How to

Returned Traveller

Dr Mike Townend

MB ChB (Hons) Diploma in Travel Medicine

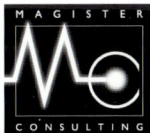

MAGISTER CONSULTING LTD

Published in the UK by
Magister Consulting Ltd
The Old Rectory, St Mary's Road
Stone, Dartford, Kent DA9 9AS

Copyright © 2004 Magister Consulting Ltd
Printed in the UK by Hartley Reproductions Ltd, Greenhithe, Kent

ISBN 1 873839 60 X

This publication reflects the views and experience of the author and not necessarily those of Magister Consulting Ltd.

Any product mentioned in the book should be used in accordance with the prescribing information prepared by the manufacturer. Neither the author nor the publisher can accept responsibility for any detrimental consequences arising from the information contained herein. Dosages given are for guidance purposes only. No sanctions or endorsements are made for any drug or compound at present under clinical investigation.

About the author

Dr Mike Townend was a GP in Cockermouth for over 25 years. He operated a Travel Clinic and Yellow Fever Vaccination Centre in his practice where he was also a GP Trainer and GP Postgraduate Tutor. His personal experience of travel ranges from travelling overland through Europe and Asia to acting as a doctor and climber with Himalayan expeditions. He also acts as a tour and trek leader in India, Nepal, Bhutan, Peru, Ecuador, Bolivia, Morocco, Thailand, Laos and Cambodia.

He was one of the first to obtain the Diploma in Travel Medicine at the University of Glasgow and now teaches on the Diploma course in addition to running a course on travel medicine at St Martin's College, Lancaster. He is a member of the Executive Committee of the British Travel Health Association, and is a member of the International Society of Travel Medicine and the International Society for Mountain Medicine.

Dr Mike Townend is the author of Travel Health for the Primary Care Team as well as chapters for two other travel health textbooks and numerous articles.

Acknowledgements

I would like to thank all those who have inspired, supported and encouraged me to pursue my interest in travel health. They include the staff, GP Registrars and partners in my former practice in Cockermouth; Dr Cameron Lockie who was largely instrumental in establishing the Glasgow Diploma in Travel Medicine which helped me to consolidate and enlarge my knowledge; Dr Eric Walker and his colleagues at the Scottish Centre for Infection and Environmental Health and all my other former teachers and fellow lecturers and tutors in Glasgow; the staff and students of St Martin's College, Lancaster; Carolyn Driver and the Executive Committee of the British Travel Health Association; Dr Steve Mellor and the Wellcome Tropical Medicine Resource for permission to use photographs from their archives; and all those travellers who travelled with me, came to me for advice before travelling or consulted me after their return.

Preface

International travel is now very much part of everyday life and, each year, more and more unusual destinations appear in the holiday brochures or travel pages of newspapers and magazines. Over the last year there have been two major incidents which have demonstrated how international travel can impact the spread of infection. Luckily, the SARS outbreak was brought under control and, so far, avian influenza has not developed into a human epidemic.

But there is no room for complacency among the healthcare professions. It is vital that a patient presenting with an acute illness is asked about their travel history and that possible 'tropical' illnesses are considered among the potential diagnoses.

Primary Care staff have many pressures placed upon them in 21st century General Practice and it is not easy to keep up-to-date in every area. This publication is ideal for such practitioners as it summarises all the key issues in a concise and easy-to-read format. While it does not set out to be a comprehensive text book, its logical format and helpful resources will be extremely useful to the busy GP or Practice Nurse.

Carolyn Driver
Independent Travel Health Specialist Nurse

Contents

Introduction

There has been an enormous growth in foreign travel over recent years. In the year 2000, 56.8 million trips abroad were made by UK residents, more than 36 million of them for holiday purposes[1]. Long-haul holiday travel has increased by almost 50% in the last five years and over 11 million such trips are now made each year from the UK. As air travel becomes a reality for more and more people, holidays in destinations such as Thailand, Kenya and Goa are now commonplace and, in the search for ever more exotic locations, areas such as the Caribbean, South America, African countries and South East Asia are rapidly becoming popular.

Ever since mankind began to journey beyond his own primitive settlements, disease has been spread by travel. From Biblical plagues to the bubonic plague of the Middle Ages and from the fall of Athens to the Spanish Conquistadors the history of the human race is littered with examples of travel-associated disease. In more recent times colonial conquests were probably responsible for the worldwide spread of cholera and, even more recently, we have seen the explosion of HIV infection across the globe.

Now that affordable air travel is within the reach of so many, the scope for the rapid spread of diseases is much greater than it has ever been[2], as was demonstrated by the spread of the severe acute respiratory syndrome (SARS)[3]. GPs and their nursing staff are becoming increasingly aware of the need to protect travelling patients before they leave. But there is a distinct possibility that, upon their return, they may be confronted with patients suffering from a wide variety of diseases not normally seen in the UK.

This book does not set out to be a textbook of tropical diseases but aims to guide the Primary Care Team through the initial stages of evaluating the problems of a patient who has returned home ill from a trip abroad.

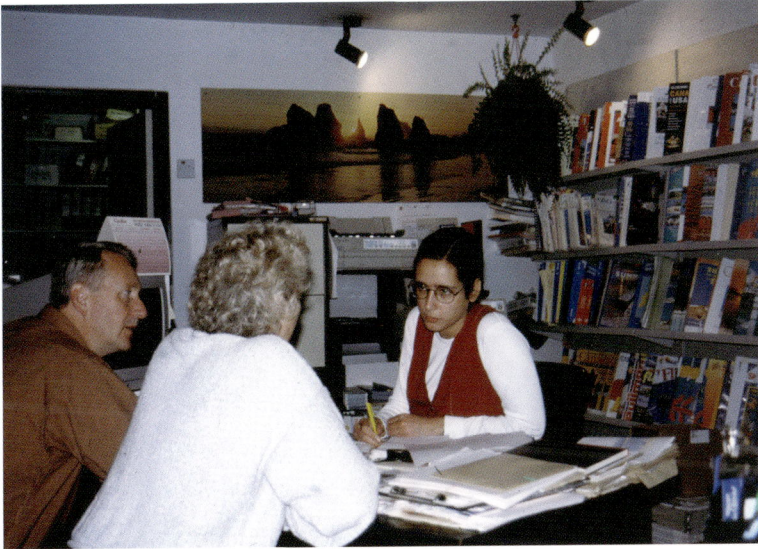

A travel agent helps her clients to choose a long-haul holiday destination

REFERENCES

1. Ahmed H, Whitmarsh A. Travel Trends. London: HMSO, 2001
2. Wilson ME. The traveller and emerging infections: sentinel, courier, transmitter. J Appl Microbiol 2003. 94 Suppl:1S-11S
3. Chan-Yeung M, Yu WC. Outbreak of severe acute respiratory syndrome in Hong Kong Special Administrative Region: case report. BMJ 2003; 326: 850-52

CHAPTER ONE

Geograhical distribution of disease

The following list is not a comprehensive account of travel-associated diseases. It is intended to illustrate the distribution of some of the health risks which exist for the traveller and to give some impression of the risks to which travellers may have been exposed.

Figures 1 to 5 show the geographical distribution of some of the more important risks[1].

- **Poliomyelitis** is spread by the faecal/oral route and is common in all countries with poor standards of hygiene.

- **Tetanus** is present worldwide but is more common in countries with poor standards of hygiene.

- **Hepatitis A** is spread by the faecal/oral route and is common in countries with poor standards of hygiene. It is a potential hazard in most countries apart from North America, northern and western Europe and Australasia. Of all the infectious diseases which can be prevented by vaccination, hepatitis A is the one most likely to be acquired by a traveller to almost all countries.

- **Hepatitis B** occurs worldwide but is more likely to occur outside those countries listed under hepatitis A above. It is spread by contact with infected blood or body fluids and procedures such as injections, major or minor surgical procedures, blood transfusions, sexual contact, tattooing and body piercing. It is considerably more infectious than HIV which is also spread by the same routes.

- **Typhoid** is also a disease spread by the faecal/oral route in countries with poor standards of hygiene, although the risk of typhoid for the traveller is 100 times less than that of hepatitis A. Most of the cases

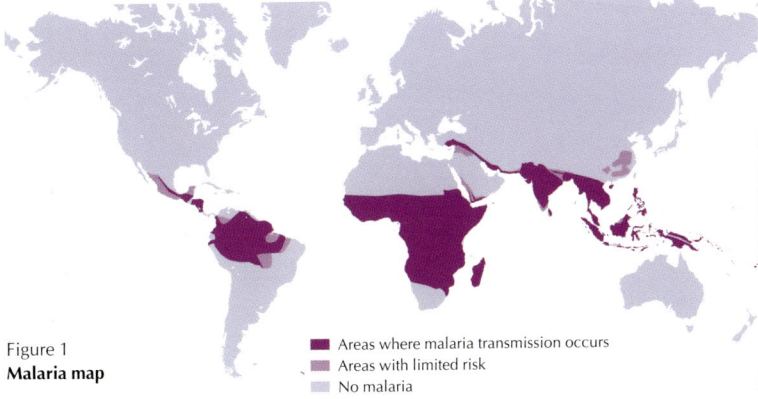

Figure 1
Malaria map

- Areas where malaria transmission occurs
- Areas with limited risk
- No malaria

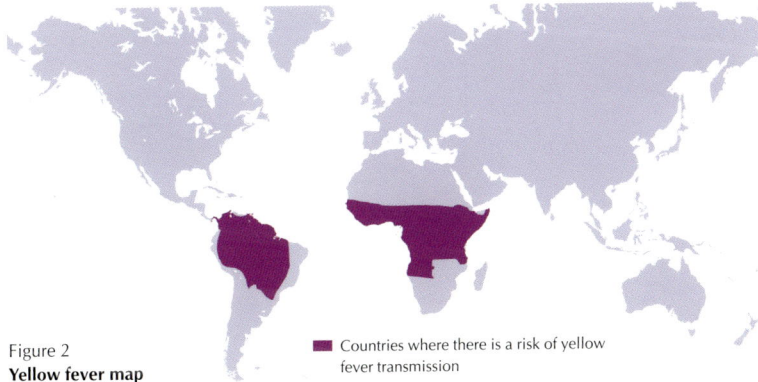

Figure 2
Yellow fever map

- Countries where there is a risk of yellow fever transmission

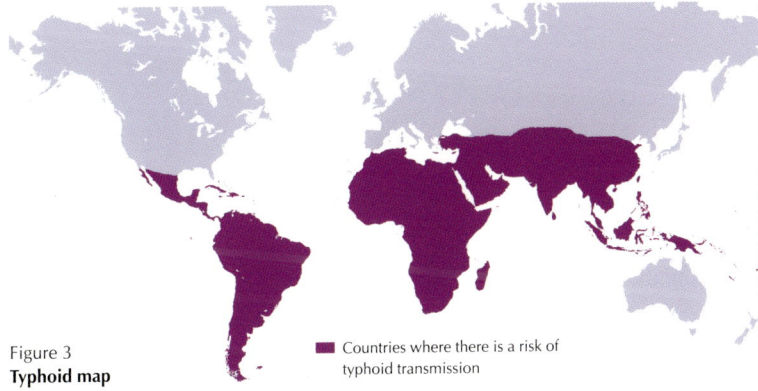

Figure 3
Typhoid map

- Countries where there is a risk of typhoid transmission

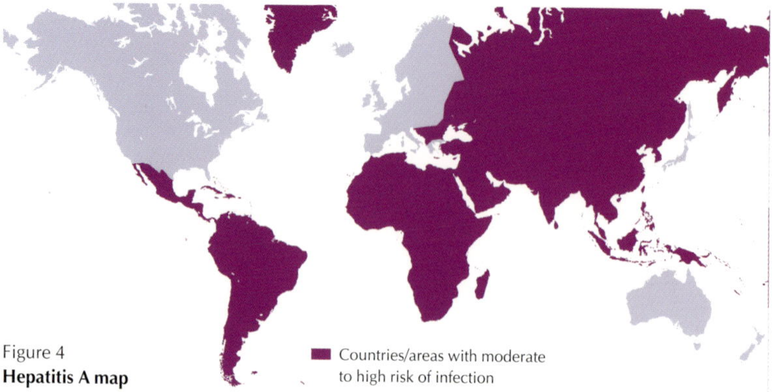

Figure 4
Hepatitis A map

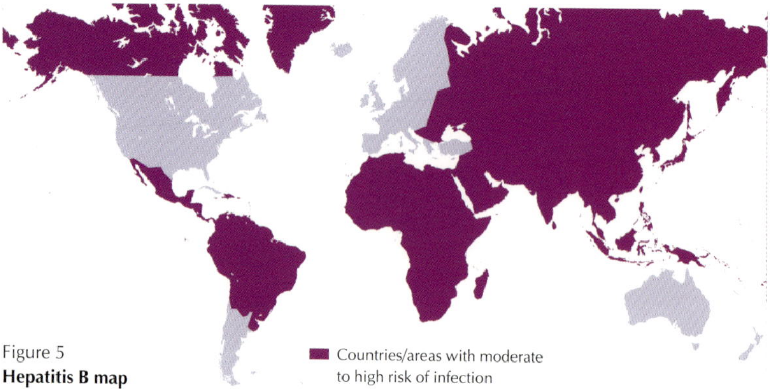

■ Countries/areas with moderate
to high risk of infection

Figure 5
Hepatitis B map

■ Countries/areas with moderate
to high risk of infection

of typhoid which are seen in the UK originate from the Indian subcontinent.

■ **Cholera** is a very low risk for travellers from the UK. It is spread in the same way as typhoid.

■ **Malaria** causes more morbidity and mortality than any other tropical infectious disease. It is widely distributed throughout sub-Saharan Africa, northern South America and Central America, the Indian sub-continent and Southeast Asia. It is spread by bites from the female Anopheles mosquito between dusk and dawn.

■ **Tuberculosis** is widespread in tropical countries and many other parts of the world but is a low risk for most UK travellers

■ **Meningitis.** Meningococcal infection is a fairly low risk for most travellers. It is most prevalent in sub-Saharan Africa.

■ **Diphtheria** is a potential risk for the unvaccinated traveller to all developing countries and to former Soviet Union countries.

■ **Dengue fever** is spread by bites from the Aedes mosquito which bites during the daytime. It is widespread throughout tropical regions of Africa, South America and Asia

■ **Yellow fever** is also spread by bites from the Aedes mosquito. It is found in northern South America and in sub-Saharan Africa.

■ **Japanese B encephalitis** is found in a band of countries from India southwards and eastwards through southeast Asia. It is spread by bites from the Culex mosquito.

■ **Tick-borne encephalitis** is found in central and eastern Europe and Scandinavia. As its name suggests, it is spread by tick bites.

■ **Schistosomiasis** is acquired by skin contact with contaminated fresh water. It is found principally in Africa, some parts of northern South America and some parts of eastern and southeastern Asia. Snails are the intermediate host for the parasites which penetrate intact skin.

■ **Filariasis** is found chiefly in Africa and in parts of Asia and South America. It is spread by bites from the Aedes, Culex or Mansonia mosquito.

■ **Trypanosomiasis** is spread by the tstete fly in Africa and by bugs in South America.

■ **Rabies.** There is a potential risk of rabies in most countries except the UK and Ireland, Scandinavia, Japan, Australia and New Zealand. It is acquired by means of a bite, scratch or possibly a lick from a small mammal. The risk for an individual traveller is low but may be more significant in Africa, India and South America.

Risk assessment for the returning traveller

As the previous section has shown, the types of diseases which the traveller may have encountered do not depend entirely on which countries he has

Dr M Townend

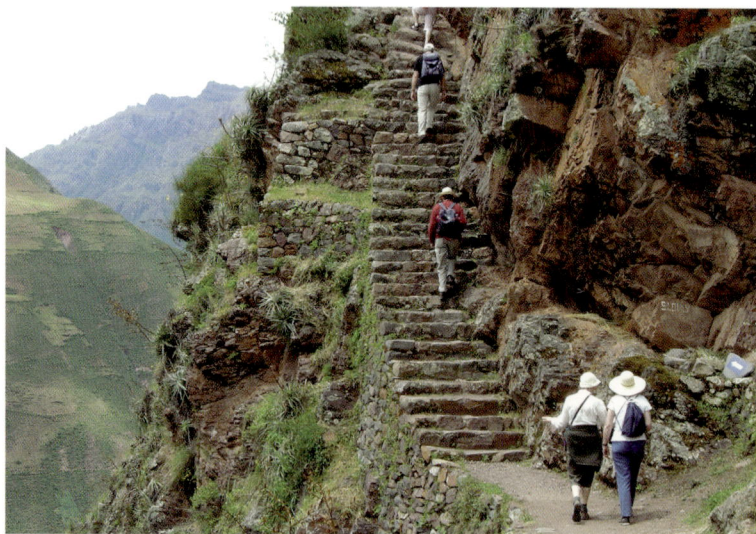

Trekking to high altitude in Peru – it is as important to know what travellers have been doing as it is to know where they have been

visited. Climate, standards of hygiene, degree of contact with local populations and the presence of suitable vectors are often more important than geography in determining risk.

In the same way that a risk assessment is needed before advising the traveller prior to travel[2], an assessment is needed of the levels of risk which the traveller has encountered during his journey when investigating the cause of his illness on his return home. A careful history of the traveller's itinerary and activities will be needed.

■ Itinerary
Disease risks may vary greatly from one part of a country to another. For example, the risk of malaria may vary from region to region or at different altitudes and the most effective type of malaria prophylaxis may also vary.

■ Length of stay
The risk of many diseases increases with increasing exposure and is therefore greater the longer the traveller's stay. Examples include hepatitis B, Japanese B encephalitis, dengue fever and filariasis.

■ Time of year
Some diseases are more prevalent at certain times of the year. For example, meningococcal disease occurs more commonly in the hot, dry season when droplet infection spreads more easily and Japanese B encephalitis occurs more commonly in the wet season.

■ Contact with soil or water
The traveller who has swum or waded in fresh water, particularly in Africa, may have acquired schistosomiasis. Strongyloides or hookworm infestation may be present in travellers who have gone barefoot or worn sandals or 'flip-flops'.

■ Contact with local people
Travellers who have been in prolonged close contact with local populations by virtue of aid, medical or teaching work or who have shared accommodation with them will have been more at risk of acquiring such diseases as tuberculosis, diphtheria or meningococcal infection.

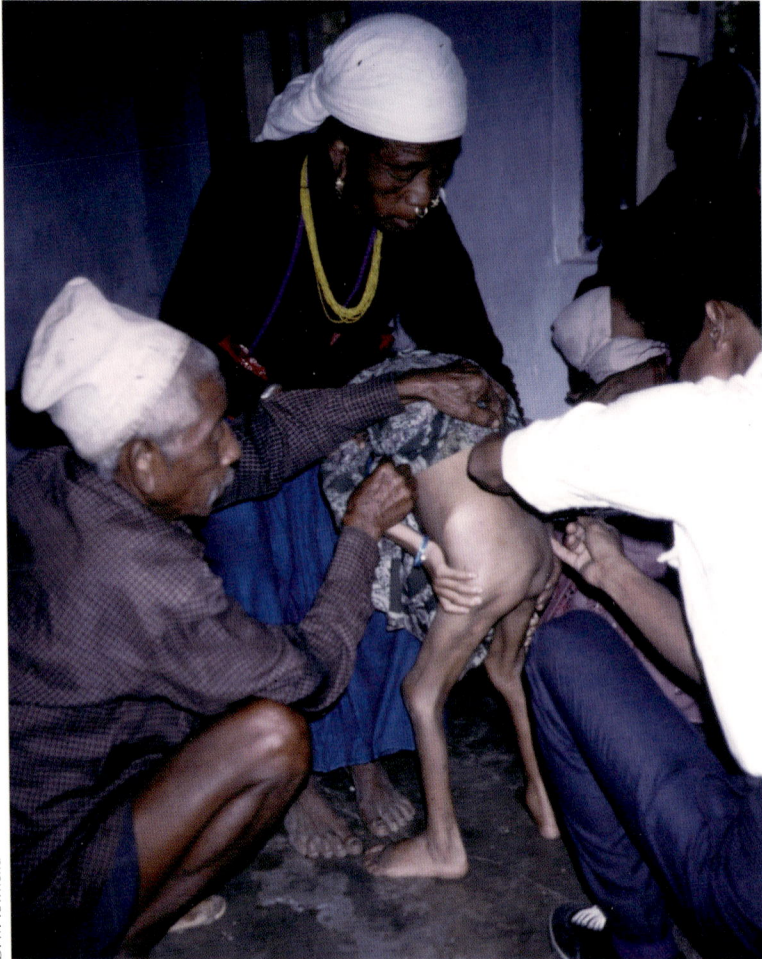

Dr M Townend

Aid workers and others in close contact with local people are more prone to droplet infection

REFERENCES

1.   World Health Organisation (www.who.int)
2.   Stringer C, Chiodinin J, Zuckerman J. International travel and health assessment. Nursing Standard 2002. 16(39):49-54

CHAPTER TWO

Evaluating the returned traveller

The traveller with a raised temperature [1,2]

Pyrexial travellers should never be assumed to have an illness such as influenza, especially if they have recently returned from a tropical country, particularly one where there is malaria and particularly from an African country. About 2,000 travellers each year return to the UK with malaria and 10 or more of them die.

Much of the serious illness which many of them suffer, and probably most of the deaths, could be avoided by earlier diagnosis and treatment. This can only occur if malaria is suspected and thick and thin blood films are examined urgently for malaria parasites. This should be done even if the traveller has taken full antimalarial drug prophylaxis and appropriate anti-mosquito precautions.

If malaria is diagnosed, or even strongly suspected, the patient should be admitted as an emergency, preferably to a specialist infectious disease unit. If malaria is excluded other clues may be obtained as to possible exposure to infection by considering:

- What areas of which countries the traveller has visited
- How long he stayed
- What kind of accommodation he used
- What activities he undertook
- How closely he mixed with local people
- What standards of food, water and personal hygiene he was able to maintain

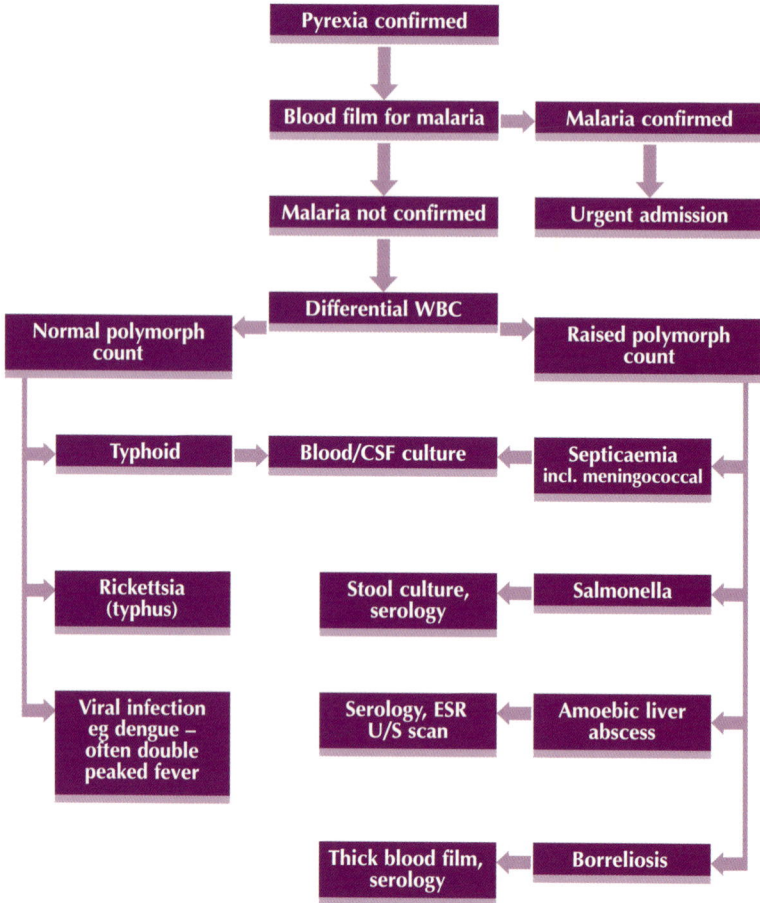

Figure 6
Initial investigation of acute pyrexia without localising signs of infection

Physical examination is important and may show:
- Localising signs of infection, eg
  - Throat infection
  - Chest signs (eg pneumonia, legionella, tuberculosis)
  - Renal or suprapubic tenderness (eg urinary tract infection)
  - Liver tenderness (eg hepatitis, amoebic liver abscess)
  - Enlarged liver and spleen (eg leishmaniasis if very large)
- Non-localising signs, eg
  - Jaundice
  - Rash
  - Lymphadenopathy
  - Enlarged spleen

A differential white cell count, which should be requested at the same time as the malaria film, is the next important investigation which may help to differentiate the causes of a pyrexia without localising signs (Figure 6). Other investigations will depend on the nature of the localising or non-localising signs observed and may include throat swabs, chest X-ray, liver function tests and a variety of serological tests.

Admission to hospital

Admission for pyrexia, preferably to a specialist infectious disease unit, is indicated if:
- Malaria is diagnosed or there is a strong suspicion of it
- The patient is very ill or prostrated by the illness
- There is a petechial rash or other evidence of bleeding. Meningococcal disease or a haemorrhagic fever may be present
- There are physical signs suggesting a tropical or other disease likely to need specialist intervention

Chronic pyrexia

A fever is usually said to be chronic if it has persisted or continued to relapse for more than two weeks. It may be caused by some of the conditions which also present acutely but there are other possible causes to add to the differential diagnosis. Once again, a differential white cell count may help towards differentiating the possible causes. Blood films for malaria must again be requested (Figure 7).

```
                    ┌─────────────────────────────┐
                    │  Chronic pyrexia confirmed  │
                    └─────────────────────────────┘
                                  │
                    ┌─────────────────────────────┐
                    │      Differential WBC       │
                    └─────────────────────────────┘
```

Normal polymorph count	Raised polymorph count
Localised tuberculosis eg pulmonary	Occult sepsis
Brucellosis	Amoebic liver abcess
Trypanosomiasis	Borreliosis (relapsing fever)
Toxoplasmosis	Cholangitis
Non-infective eg auto-immune	

Reduced polymorph count	Raised eosinophil count
Malaria	Schistosomiasis
Miliary tuberculosis	Filariasis
Visceral leishmanisasis	Larva migrans (eg toxocara)
Brucellosis	

Figure 7

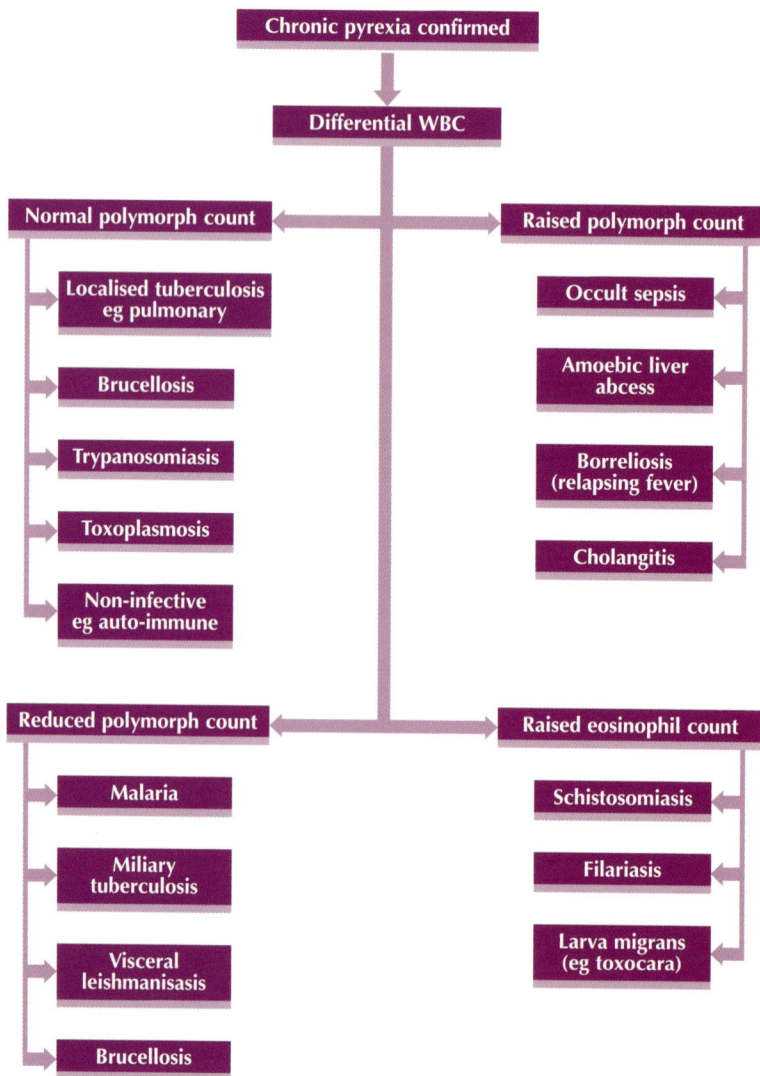

Initial investigation of a traveller with chronic pyrexia

Whatever the suspicions raised following a white cell count it is likely that the GP will need to discuss further investigation with an infectious disease specialist or refer or admit the patient, depending on the nature of the suspicion and on how ill the patient is. The patient's travel history may again provide clues to the risks to which he has been exposed. Further tests may include:

- Blood films for malaria, filariasis or borreliosis
- Liver function tests
- Ultrasound liver scan
- Serological tests
- Urine test or rectal biopsy for schistosomiasis

The traveller with diarrhoea [3, 4]

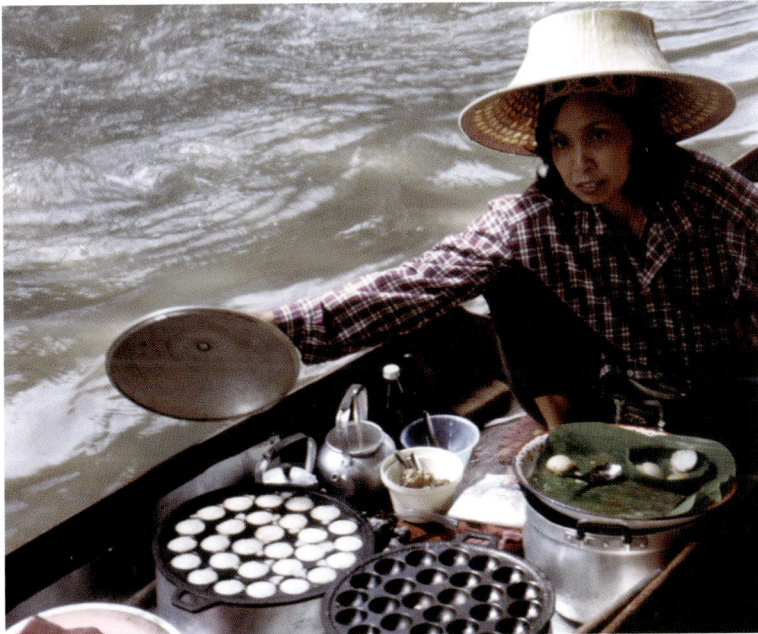

Dr M Townend

A floating market in Thailand – food from stalls such as this is a frequent source of diarrhoeal illness

Diarrhoea is the symptom most likely to be experienced by travellers to developing or low-income countries, with a risk of 50% or more in some countries. Causative organisms include bacteria such as E. coli; Shigella spp.; Salmonella spp.; Campylobacter; bacterial toxins from organisms such as Staph. aureus and Clostridium; viruses such as Rotavirus and Norwalk virus; protozoa such as Entamoeba and Giardia; flukes such as Schistosoma and worms, particularly Strongyloides.

Diarrhoea may also be caused by multi-organ diseases such as malaria and Legionella infection. Blood films for malaria are an essential part of the investigation of any traveller with diarrhoea and pyrexia who has recently returned from a malarial country.

Bacterial and viral infections are likely to cause acute and frequent diarrhoea, while protozoal infections are more likely to cause a less acute onset with a lower stool frequency and a more chronic course. A traveller who has been exposed to poor standards of food and water hygiene and who returns home with chronic diarrhoea and weight loss may have a Cyclospora infection. If, in addition, he has offensive flatus or belching he may be infected with Giardia. A long-term traveller or expatriate worker with chronic malabsorptive diarrhoea may have tropical sprue.

The presence of blood in the stools or the presence of pyrexia are important factors in differentiating possible causes of diarrhoea (Figure 8). Investigation should include:

- Blood films for malaria in all patients with pyrexia and diarrhoea who have been to a malarial area
- Stool culture. If amoebiasis is a possibility the stool should be examined as soon as possible after it has been passed
- Differential white cell count. Bacterial infections may produce a raised polymorphonuclear leucocyte count, although S. typhi does not do so. Lymphocytosis may suggest a viral infection and eosinophilia will suggest the presence of intestinal parasites or schistosomiasis
- Serological tests for salmonella spp.

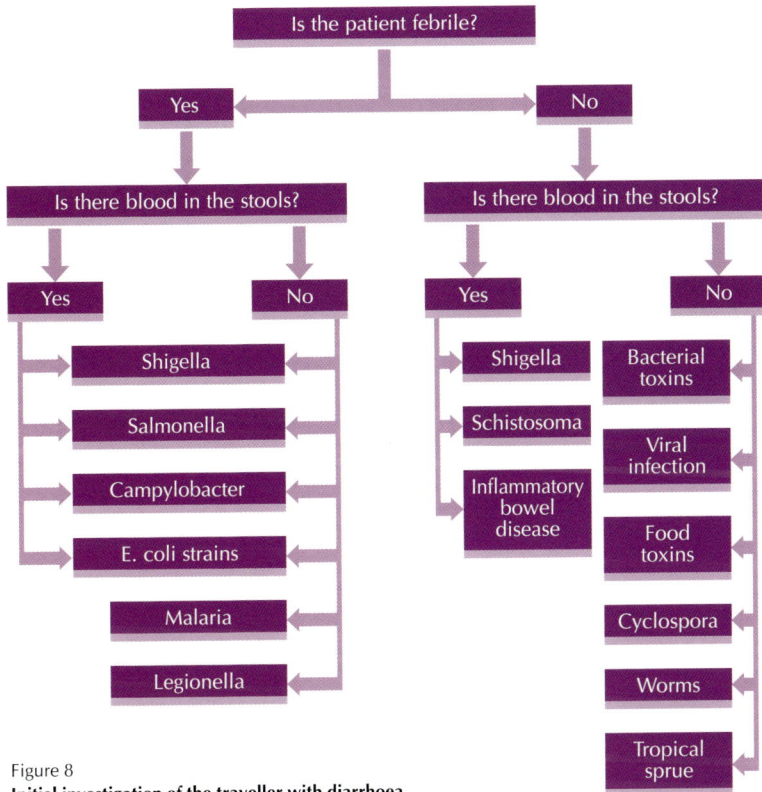

Figure 8
Initial investigation of the traveller with diarrhoea

Referral to hospital

Referral, ideally to a specialised infectious diseases unit, should be considered if:

- The patient has severe diarrhoea with potential or actual dehydration
- Malaria is suspected. Do not wait for the result of investigations as delay can be fatal
- Blood in the stools or other clinical features suggest the presence of a tropical infection or other condition likely to need specialist intervention

Treatment of diarrhoea

- Rehydration is of the greatest importance, particularly if diarrhoea is severe
- Admission to hospital if rehydration cannot be achieved orally, eg if there is associated vomiting
- Antibacterial drugs such as ciprofloxacin 500mg twice a day should be started if the patient is ill and pyrexial without waiting for the result of a stool culture
- Antidiarrhoeal drugs such as loperamide may be helpful to reduce stool frequency

The traveller with jaundice

Malaria
Any traveller who has returned from a malarial country who is ill, pyrexial and jaundiced must have blood films examined for malaria.

Hepatitis
The most likely cause of jaundice in a returning traveller is hepatitis. In the case of hepatitis A, the vaccine-preventable disease most likely to be encountered by travellers[5], the patient is likely to have experienced pyrexia, headache, malaise and aches and pains before the jaundice becomes evident and may well feel much better by the time jaundice appears.

Children may have a mild or even sub-clinical illness without jaundice. The clinical picture in other forms of hepatitis is similar but the incubation period of hepatitis B is much longer and may extend to many weeks. There may be a history of medical or other invasive procedures or of sexual exposure. Hepatitis E may have been acquired, particularly in the Indian subcontinent, by the same faecal-oral route as hepatitis A and hepatitis C may have been acquired in similar ways to hepatitis B

Leptospirosis
Immersion in fresh water contaminated by rat urine as a result of swimming or other water sports or during cave exploration may lead to leptospirosis. A flu-like illness with muscle pains, diarrhoea and conjunctivitis, it may lead to jaundice.

Investigation of jaundice
- Blood films for malaria
- Differential white cell count
- Liver function tests
- Serological tests for hepatitis A, B, C and E and leptospirosis

Treatment of jaundice
Patients with hepatitis A usually recover without serious sequelae though fulminant hepatitis may occur with any type of viral hepatitis. Leptospirosis responds to appropriate antibiotic treatment.

Referral to hospital
The seriously-ill jaundiced patient will need hospital admission, preferably to a specialist infectious disease unit, whatever diagnosis is suspected.

The traveller with a rash[6]

Bites
Apart from sunburn the most frequent cause of a skin problem with which a returned traveller may present is insect bites. Allergic reactions to bites are common and may be small and intensely itchy papules or larger areas of swelling and erythema. Infection from scratching often occurs and may result in pustules or enlargement of regional lymph nodes.

Bites from flying insects are usually found on exposed areas of skin or around the ankles and animal fleas bite on areas of contact with the animal, again often around the ankles, or on areas of contact with furnishings which are infested from contact with animals. Flea bites often occur in groups in a linear distribution. They are more likely to occur in backpackers or low budget travellers.

Calamine lotion may relieve itching temporarily or oral antihistamine drugs may be needed. Topical or systemic antibacterial therapy, for example with flucloxacillin, may be needed for infected bites.

Evaluation of rashes in the returned traveller

Some of the types of rash which returning travellers may present are as follows, though this is a far from complete list:

- Itchy papular rash on exposed areas or around ankles, with or without secondary infection: insect bites
- Transient itchy rash a few hours after bathing or swimming in fresh water, especially in Africa: schistosomiasis ('swimmer's itch')
- Erythematous rash spreading out from the site of a tick bite, with or without flu-like symptoms (erythema chronicum migrans): Lyme disease
- Migrating, irregular, linear, itchy skin lesion, especially after skin contact with soil or sand (erythema chronicum migrans)
- Indolent ulcer on exposed area of skin: cutaneous leishmaniasis or cutaneous diphtheria
- Irregular streaky or blistering lesions: contact with plant toxins or irritants

Treatment of skin lesions

The treatment of bites has already been discussed. Tetracycline antibiotics are indicated to prevent further development of Lyme disease and a single dose of

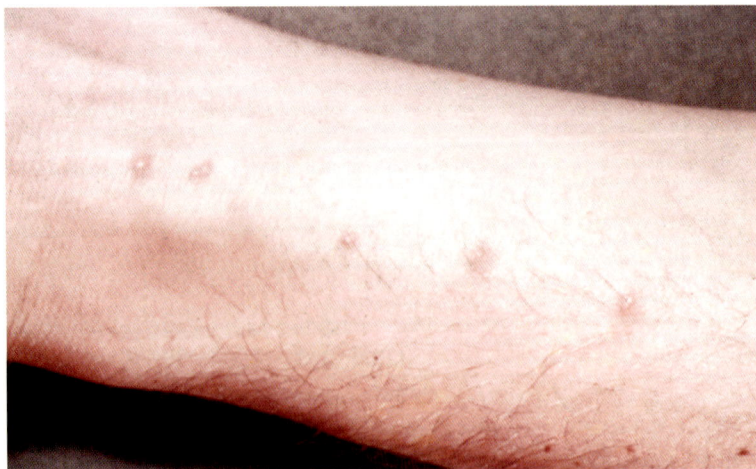

Wellcome Tropical Medicine Resource and Centers for Disease Control

Swimmer's itch, produced by initial infection with schistosomiasis

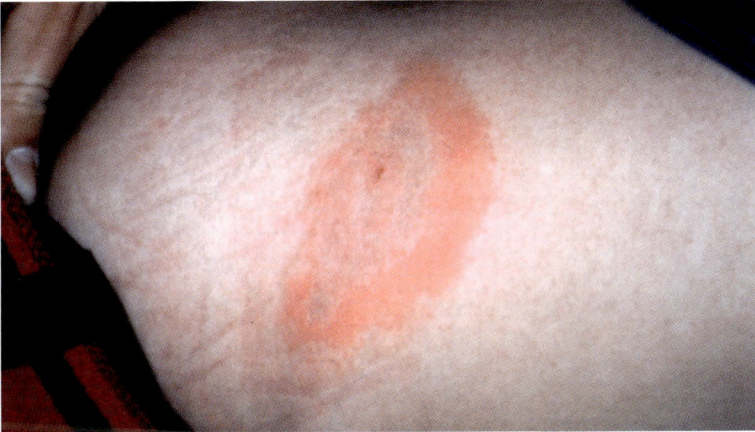

Erythema chronicum migrans, the skin lesion of Lyme disease following a tick bite

Wellcome Tropical Medicine Resource and Royal Army Medical College

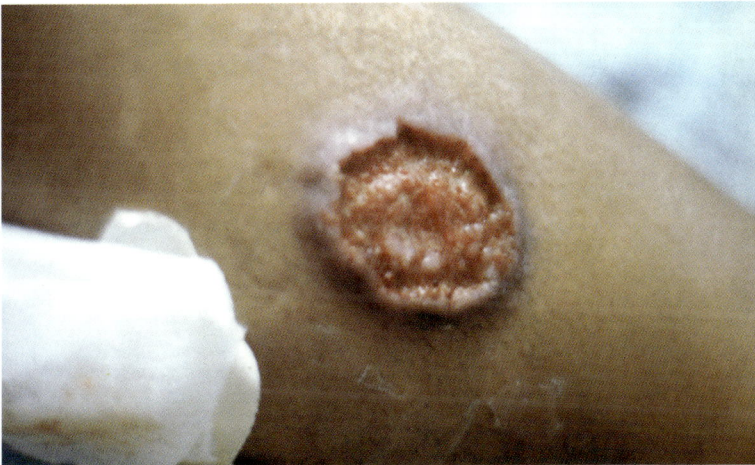

Skin ulceration caused by cutaneous leishmaniasis

Wellcome Tropical Medicine Resource

praziquantel is effective for the early stages of schistosomiasis. Cutaneous larva migrans may be self-limiting as it is caused by hookworm larvae which are not usually pathogenic for man and which eventually die after failing to find a resting place in an inappropriate host. It can be treated with albendazole, especially if there are numerous larvae present

Post travel screening [7]

Most travellers who return home with health problems will have symptoms of illness. Routine screening of returned travellers is therefore likely to be unproductive and in most cases is unnecessary. A possible exception to this may be the long-term expatriate who has lived or worked in a tropical country and/or a country with a high risk of parasitic or other chronic diseases which may not present with acute or dramatic symptoms. For example, infestation with the intestinal worm Strongyloides may persist for many years and may begin to cause symptoms of diarrhoea or abdominal discomfort after months or years.

If screening is thought necessary in the asymptomatic or minimally symptomatic returned traveller it should include:

- Full blood count and differential white cell count including eosinophils
- Stool microscopy and culture
- Chest X-ray if there has been a substantial risk of exposure to tuberculosis
- Serological or other specific tests for any diseases from which the traveller has been at particularly high risk after taking a careful history of the countries in which he has lived and the activities which he has undertaken. Hepatitis B seropositivity is sometimes seen in expatriates and/or their families after long stays abroad and a serological test should be included in their screening

Referral to a specialist unit is advisable if any of these tests give positive results.

Post travel debriefing

Long-term expatriates and aid workers will have undergone a process of adjustment of their values and social customs to life and work in a very different environment. This may sometimes have been a long and painful process both physically and psychologically. On their return home they are faced with a readjustment to a familiar environment and way of life which may well be at least as difficult or, in many cases, more difficult than their first adjustment.

Life in the home country may have moved on in ways which they do not understand and their family and friends may have changed during their absence. In addition, the travellers themselves will inevitably have been changed by their experiences and many of the trappings of life at home may seem trivial or irrelevant in the light of these experiences.

Many agencies which send workers abroad, eg to aid projects, include a debriefing period on returning home as part of their overall package but many others do not. Those who are finding the process of readjustment difficult should be referred to a counsellor or to a specialist post travel counselling service. Inter Health and Care for Mission provide such a service for those who have worked abroad for aid agencies or Christian missions.

REFERENCES

1. Felton JM, Bryceson AD. Fever in the returning traveller. Brit J Hosp Med 1996. 55(11):705-11
2. Suh KN, Kozarsky PE, Keystone JS. Evaluation of fever in the returned traveller. Med Clin N America 1999. 83(4):997-1017
3. Ellis C. Diarrhoea in the returned traveller. Practitioner 1996. 240(1560):188-92
4. Farthing MJ. Travellers' diarrhoea. Gut 1994. 35(1):1.4
5. Steffen R. Hepatitis A in travellers: the European experience. J Inf Dis 1995. 171 Suppl 1:S24-8
6. McCarron B. Diagnosing imported rashes and skin lesions. Practitioner 1998. 242(1586):366-8
7. Churchill DR, Chiodini Pl, McAdam KP. Screening the returned traveller. Brit Med Bull 1993. 49(2):465-74

CHAPTER THREE

Travel associated diseases

Gastrointestinal diseases

Travellers' diarrhoea is the condition most likely to afflict travellers from developed to less well developed countries. Depending on where they have been, 20 to 50% or possibly more of travellers returning from such countries will have had at least one episode of diarrhoea while abroad and some of them will still have symptoms on their return home.

Causes of diarrhoea may include an unfamiliar diet or changes in 'normal' gut flora, but most are caused by infection by pathogenic organisms:

■ Enterotoxic E. coli and viruses such as rotavirus and Norwalk virus are common causes.

■ Other bacterial causes include various species of Salmonella and Shigella as well as Campylobacter.

■ Bacterial toxins from Staph. aureus or Clostridium spp. may be implicated.

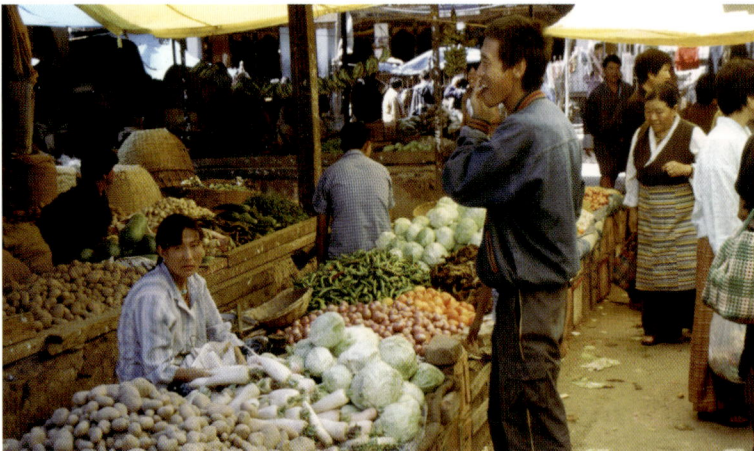

Dr M Townend

A Bhutanese fruit and vegetable market – eating unpeeled fruit may be a cause of travellers' diarrhoea

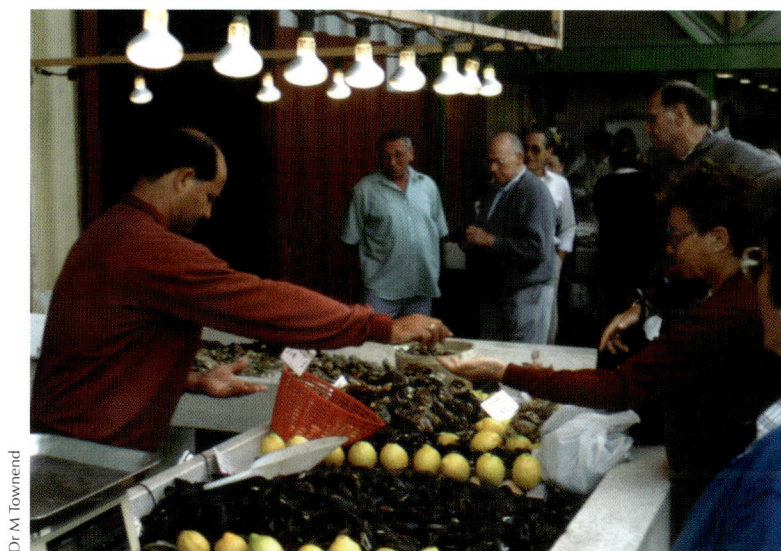

Dr M Townend

Shellfish, especially if uncooked, are a fertile source of gastrointestinal infection

- Bacterial or viral infections are likely to be acute and many of them will have resolved or been treated before the traveller returns home. But they may still be symptomatic on returning.
- Protozoal infections such as Entamoeba histolytica, Giardia or Cyclospora are likely to cause more persistent and less dramatic or frequent diarrhoea and may well present as chronic diarrhoea on returning home, possibly with weight loss if they are of long standing.
- Chronic diarrhoea and loss of weight may also be caused by tropical sprue in which there is intestinal malabsorption and, coincidentally, some travellers may have developed problems not associated with travel or infection such as inflammatory bowel disease.
- Heavy infestation with worms such as Strongyloides may occasionally cause diarrhoea in returned travellers, particularly after long stays in conditions of poor hygiene.
- Diarrhoea may persist after an infective illness in the form of a post-infective irritable bowel syndrome but this possibility should not detract from the necessity of investigating diarrhoea fully.

Transmission of travellers' diarrhoea is by and large by the faecal/oral route and is associated with poor standards of food and water hygiene in a country and/or poor personal hygiene on the part of food handlers. Contaminated food and drinking water are the main vehicles but ice in drinks and swallowing water in showers or swimming pools or cleaning teeth with tap water may result in infection.

Clinical features apart from diarrhoea may include systemic symptoms such as fever and symptoms localised to the bowel such as blood in the stools.

- The presence of fever suggests a bacterial or viral infection but the possibility of a multi-organ disease such a malaria or Legionella infection should be borne in mind.
- Diarrhoea without fever is seen in protozoal infections and toxic diarrhoea as well as inflammatory bowel disease and tropical sprue.
- The presence of blood in the stools suggests the presence of infection which has invaded and damaged the bowel mucosa, such as Shigella, Salmonella, Campylobacter, Entamoeba, invasive strains of E. coli or schistosomiasis, or of inflammatory bowel disease.
- Watery diarrhoea without blood suggests infection with pathogenic E. coli, viral agents or cyclospora. Profuse, prostrating, watery diarrhoea suggests cholera, though this is seldom seen in UK-based travellers.
- Profuse, offensive flatus or belching may be seen with giardiasis.

Investigation of diarrhoea is not always necessary as it may be self-limiting. Severe or persistent diarrhoea should be investigated as should diarrhoea accompanied by the passage of blood. Initial investigation has been discussed in Chapter 2.

- ***Stool testing.*** At least three stool specimens taken on different days must be examined before infection can be excluded and the stools should be examined as soon as possible after being passed if Entamoeba infection is suspected. Stools should be examined by someone experienced in microscopy of tropical infections as non-pathogenic species of amoeba may be present coincidentally and a mistaken diagnosis of amoebiasis may be made.

- ***Serological tests*** are available for Salmonella typhi and paratyphi, amoebiasis and schistosomiasis.

■ **Further investigation** may involve tests for malabsorption, endoscopy and rectal biopsy and specialist referral will be needed if invasive infection, malabsorption or inflammatory bowel disease are suspected.

■ Do not forget the possibility of malaria or Legionella.

Treatment of diarrhoea may be started without investigation or before the results of tests are available.

■ **Glucose/electrolyte solution** replaces lost fluid and helps to reverse the secretion of fluid by the intestinal mucosa by promoting absorption of glucose and sodium and, indirectly, of water. Oral rehydration is particularly important for children and the elderly. Otherwise, copious fluids containing a small amount of salt together with easily absorbed carbohydrate foods such as boiled rice, potatoes and white bread may suffice.

■ **Antidiarrhoeal drugs** are of most use when the traveller is actually travelling as increased stool frequency can be a great problem. They should not be used for children and find their greatest use in adults who have frequent stools without the passage of blood.

■ **Antimicrobial drugs** may be used for the treatment of diarrhoea, particularly if it is persistent for several days and/or associated with a raised temperature. It is not necessary to wait for the results of a stool culture. A quinolone such as **ciprofloxacin** 500mg twice a day for 5 to 7 days will be effective for most intestinal bacterial pathogens. There is now evidence that a single dose of 500mg is effective in a high proportion of cases of travellers' diarrhoea. **Co-trimoxazole** is an alternative choice but its side-effect profile is less favourable. **Metronidazole** or **tinidazole** are effective against Entamoeba and Giardia.

Intestinal parasites are common in the indigenous population of developing countries. They may be acquired by travellers, particularly those who are exposed to a higher level of risk by virtue of residence or prolonged stays, remote or rural travel or living in conditions similar to those of the local population. They are usually acquired by the faecal/oral route from eggs or larvae in contaminated food or water, although some may be acquired by penetration of intact human skin. Infestation is therefore possible in travellers whose itinerary or living conditions have fitted the above profile or who have been in the habit of walking barefoot. Many parasites produce few or no symptoms, especially if the numbers present in the gut are relatively small.

Metazoa

■ **Roundworms** (Ascaris lumbricoides) are acquired by the faecal/oral route by swallowing active embryonated eggs. Larvae are then produced in the gut and migrate in the blood to the lungs where they increase in size. From the lung they migrate up the trachea and are then swallowed to reach their habitat in the gut. During their passage through the lung they may produce cough and wheeze and possibly fever, and examination of the blood may show eosinophilia. Chest X-ray may show scattered areas of shadowing. Otherwise, symptoms are uncommon unless there is a heavy worm-load in the gut, when discomfort or colicky pain may occur and even intestinal obstruction. Worms may appear in the stools or be vomited up, when their large size may cause alarm and eggs can be found in a stool specimen. Treatment is with a variety of anthelmintic drugs including piperazine and mebendazole.

■ **Strongyloides** is acquired from faecal contamination of soil by penetration of intact human skin by filariform larvae which enter the lungs via the blood. As with roundworms they then migrate up the trachea to be swallowed and reach their gut habitat. Larvae produced in the gut may penetrate the gut wall and reach the lungs, perpetuating the cycle of reproduction within the host. Clinical features of infection may include a transient itchy rash at the point of entry and occasionally cough or wheeze similar to that seen in Ascaris infestation during lung migration. Abdominal pain and diarrhoea may occur and with a heavy worm-load malabsorption may occur. Because of the process of auto-reinfestation, symptoms may continue to recur for many years. Eggs can be found in a stool specimen and eosinophilia may be found.

■ **Tapeworms** (Taenia solium or T. saginata from pork or beef respectively) may be acquired by swallowing encysted larvae in the form of cysticerci in undercooked meat. The larvae ultimately develop into adult worms composed of many segments which may grow to a length of as much as several metres. T. solium may also be acquired by swallowing eggs which produce cysticerci. This may then lead to cysticercosis in which encysted larvae or cysticerci are found in skin, muscles or in the brain. Diagnosis often follows the passage of tapeworm segments which may continue to be motile after being passed either in a stool or by emerging of their own accord from the anus. Treatment of either species is best carried out with niclosamide.

■ *Hydatid disease* is caused by human infestation with the dog tapeworm which results in the presence of hydatid cysts in the liver, lungs or elsewhere. It may be detected by serological tests.

■ *Hookworm* (Ankylostoma or Necator spp.) is acquired from faecal contamination of soil by penetration of intact human skin by filariform larvae. Once again, migration to the lung occurs followed by the larvae being swallowed and reaching the gut, though some species may reach the gut direct. In the gut the larvae attach themselves to the wall of the small intestine and feed on blood. Clinical features may include an itchy rash at the site of penetration and cough or wheeze during lung migration. Otherwise, the principal manifestation, especially with a heavy worm-load, is anaemia. Diagnosis is made by finding eggs in a stool specimen and an iron deficiency anaemia. Mebendazole may be used for treatment of hookworm although a variety of other drugs may be used. Anaemia requires treatment with oral iron.

■ Larvae of the dog hookworm may penetrate human skin but are unable to find a definitive habitat. They 'wander' about the skin leaving a serpiginous and intensely itchy track known as cutaneous larva migrans. Thiabendazole is effective in treatment.

■ *Whipworm* (Trichuris) is acquired by the faecal/oral route by swallowing active embryonated eggs. There is no lung migration stage. Clinical features may include diarrhoea, possibly with the passage of blood and, with heavy infestation, rectal prolapse. Anaemia may also occur. Diagnosis is made by finding eggs in a stool specimen. Mebendazole or albendazole may be used for treatment.

Protozoa

■ *Amoebiasis* (Entamoeba histolytica) is acquired by the faecal/oral route by ingestion of cysts in contaminated food or water. The resulting vegetative forms of amoeba may be completely asymptomatic but may become invasive. Ulceration of the mucosa results and the amoebae ingest red blood cells. The resulting dysentery may last for several weeks and then subside again into vegetative co-existence, only to relapse again in the future. Clinical features include diarrhoea with the passage of blood but without fever, and complications may include haemorrhage or bowel perforation and occasionally bowel necrosis with ileus. Diarrhoea is usually not of acute onset or as frequent as that which occurs with bacterial infections and often involves the passage of blood. Amoebic liver abscess may occur as an early or late complication, with hepatic pain and tenderness, hepatomegaly, fever and possibly basal lung signs. Diagnosis of amoebiasis is made by microscopy of a freshly passed stool specimen. Confusion may arise from the presence of non-pathogenic strains of amoeba or of E. histolytica which is not currently invasive. Invasive amoebae will be seen to contain ingested red blood cells in a freshly passed stool. Amoebic liver abscess may be diagnosed by serological tests, a raised polymorphonuclear leucocyte count and an ultrasound liver scan. Intestinal amoebiasis and liver abscess are treated with metronidazole and diloxanide.

■ *Giardiasis* (Giardia lamblia) is acquired by the faecal/oral route by ingestion of cysts from contaminated food or water. Diarrhoea is not necessarily acute in onset, but may be, and again is not excessively frequent. It may be accompanied by the passing of offensive wind upwards or downwards and there may be a feeling of distension or bloating. Diagnosis is usually made by the finding of cysts in a stool specimen.

Diseases spread by insect vectors

Malaria

In terms of illness and death worldwide, malaria is the most important of the tropical diseases. It is caused by infection with parasites of the genus Plasmodium, the four species concerned being P. falciparum, P. vivax, P. ovale and P. malariae. Female Anopheles mosquitoes inject sporozooites into the human from which they take a blood meal and a complex life cycle follows in the human host involving stages in the liver and blood.

Symptoms occur when infected blood cells rupture to release showers of merozoites. This process occurs in cycles which give the classical periodicity of fever but the periodicity said to be typical of a particular type of malaria ('tertian' or 'quartan') is not always seen. Malaria cannot be excluded simply because there is not a peak in the fever every third or fourth day. In addition to presenting as a fever, malaria may also present with diarrhoea or jaundice.

■ *P. vivax and P. ovale* parasites may form a 'hypnozoite' stage in the liver in which they remain dormant for weeks or even months before becoming active and causing fever. A diagnosis of malaria must always be considered in any patient who has travelled to a malarial country in the last six or even 12 months and who has a feverish illness.

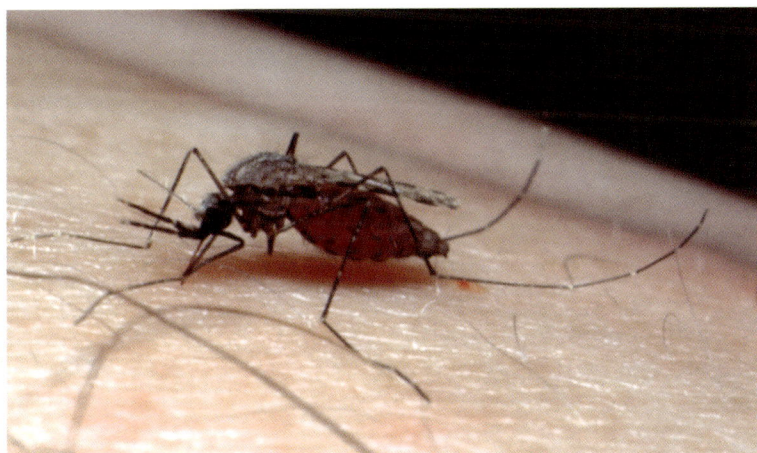

Wellcome Tropical Medicine Resource and Dr A Stich

Malaria parasites are transmitted to humans by the bites of the female Anopheles mosquito

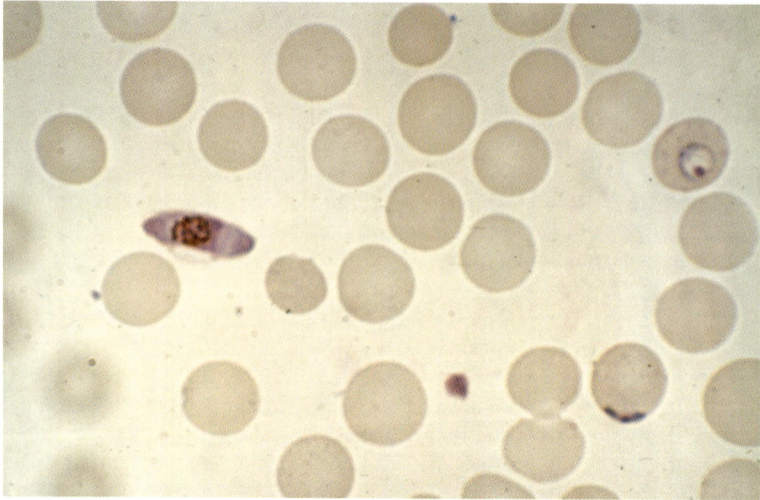

Wellcome Tropical Medicine Resource

A thin blood film showing the presence of Plasmodium falciparum

- *P. falciparum* causes a much more serious and possibly fatal disease. Disruption of red cells in this type of malaria occurs deep in the capillaries in the tissues rather than in the superficial circulation as it does in other types. A severe multi-organ disease can follow involving the gastrointestinal tract, liver, lungs, kidneys or brain. Diarrhoea, jaundice, pneumonia, nephritis and meningoencephalitis may all be seen as presentations of falciparum malaria or may occur if there is a delay in making a diagnosis.

- *Diagnosis* of malaria is made by examining a thick blood film, which increases the chances of seeing parasites, and a thin blood film in which the type of parasite is more easily determined. It is not necessary to wait for a specific stage in the illness in order to take a blood specimen but the specimen should be examined as a matter of urgency whatever the time of day or night and the report telephoned as soon as it is available. Further specimens must be submitted if the test is negative but a strong suspicion exists.

- *Preventive measures* including the use of antimalarial drugs, avoiding exposing the skin unduly, using insect repellents and sleeping under a mosquito net reduce the likelihood of infection but do not eliminate it. Malaria must be considered as a cause of fever or other symptoms even if all necessary precautions have been taken.

■ **Treatment** of malaria should be undertaken in a specialist infectious disease unit. Admission should be requested if malaria is strongly suspected or if investigation of a fever suggests it. For drug doses for both prophylaxis and treatment see Chapter 4.

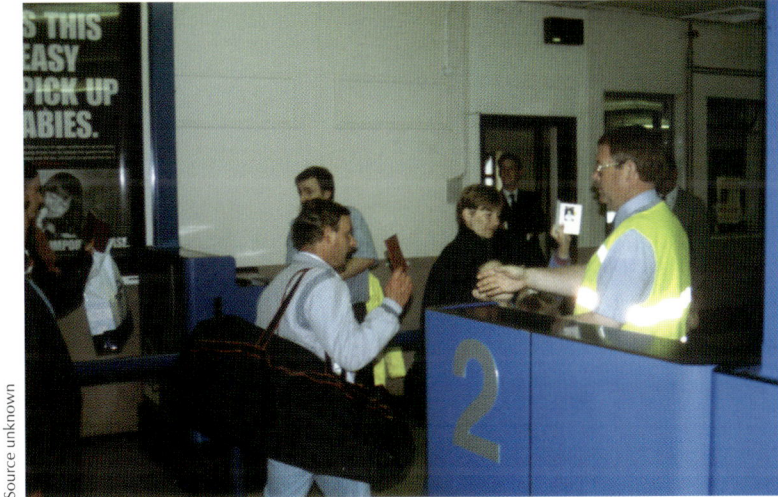

Immigrants are at particular risk of malaria when returning home to visit relatives

■ **Immunity to malaria** is acquired only after living in a malarial country for at least 10 to 15 years. Expatriates serving lesser terms abroad will need to take preventive measures. Immigrants to non-malarial countries rapidly lose their immunity and they and their families are at particular risk from malaria as they are unlikely to perceive a risk from a disease against which they took no precautions in their country of origin.

Malaria in the returned traveller

- Suspect malaria in anyone with a fever who has travelled to a malarial area in the last six to 12 months.

- Suspect malaria in patients with diarrhoea or jaundice if they have visited a malarial area.

- Do not expect to see a characteristic pattern of fever.

- Investigate urgently any suspicion of malaria by thick and thin blood films.

- Do not delay investigation by waiting for a specific stage in the fever.

- Do not assume that taking antimalarial drugs or other precautions excludes the possibility of malaria.

- Beware of malaria in immigrants and their families after a visit to their country of origin.

- Admit to a specialist unit if malaria is suspected.

Arthropod-borne viruses (Arboviruses)

- *Yellow fever* originally arose as a viral infection in monkeys. It is found only in tropical regions of Africa and South America. The vector is the Aedes mosquito which is capable of transmitting the virus to humans by means of its bites and from human to human. It is a serious illness and after an initial period of fever, aches, pains and headaches it may then produce jaundice, bleeding and progressive hepatic and renal impairment. Diagnosis may be made by viral studies and serological tests but admission to hospital will be needed in view of the severity of the illness. There is no definitive treatment.

- *Dengue* is widespread in tropical regions and is one of the most frequently occurring tropical diseases. In travellers it is more likely to occur during long stays abroad which increase the risk of exposure to infected mosquitoes. A viral infection which is spread by the bites of Aedes mosquitoes, it presents as a severe flu-like illness with marked muscular pains ('break-bone fever'). As with some other viral fevers there may be a 'double hump' with temporary remission of fever during its course. Dengue haemorrhagic fever is a serious complication. Rare in travellers, it is more common in children and appears to be associated with previous infection with dengue or other viruses. Diagnosis is made by viral studies or serological tests. There is no definitive treatment.

- **_Japanese B encephalitis_** is a viral infection spread by Culex mosquitoes. It is found throughout southern and southeastern Asia but no longer in Japan. It is found mostly in rural areas in the wet season where there are rice paddies in which the mosquitoes breed and where there are domesticated animals such as pigs which act as an intermediate host. It may be suspected in unvaccinated travellers whose itinerary fits this profile. It presents with fever, headache and vomiting and signs of central nervous involvement follow. Admission to hospital and lumbar puncture will be needed to establish the diagnosis.

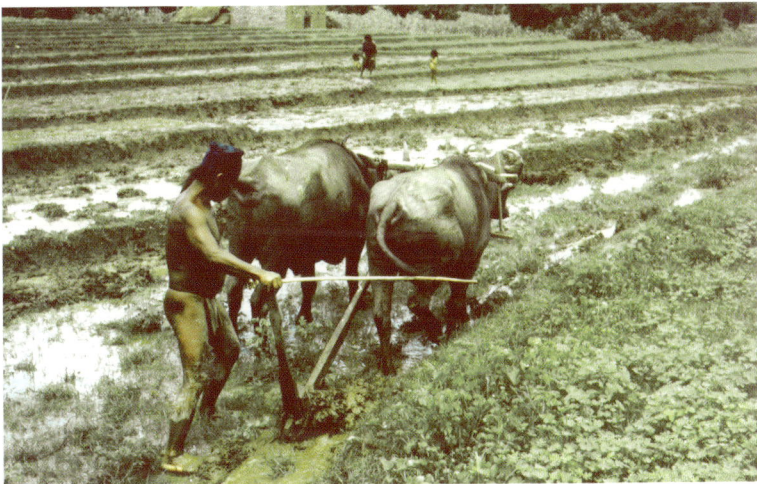

Dr M Townend

Japanese B encephalitis is most likely to occur in the wet season in rice growing areas

Other diseases spread by insects

■ **Filariasis** is transmitted from human to human by the bites of various types of mosquito. It is found in Africa, Asia and South America. Microfilariae, taken up by the mosquito from an infected human, develop into larvae which are then injected into another human host. These filariform larvae enter the lymphatic system and, after a latent period of months, intermittent lymphangitis is seen. In indigenous populations this may lead to lymphoedema and hypertrophy typical of elephantiasis although this is rarely seen in travellers. Release of microfilariae into the bloodstream may take place during the day or the night, depending on the species of filaria involved. Diagnosis depends on finding microfilariae in the blood at the appropriate time although serological tests are also available.

■ **Leishmaniasis** in its cutaneous form is found in Central and South America, around the Mediterranean, in the Middle East and in parts of Africa and Asia. The insect vector is the female sandfly. Although there are several clinical manifestations, the most usual form found in travellers is an indolent ulcer, usually on an exposed area of skin.

■ **Visceral leishmaniasis** (kala-azar) is found in similar areas of the world and is characterised by intermittent fever followed by considerable enlargement of the liver and spleen. It is uncommon in travellers.

■ **Trypanosomiasis.** African trypanosomiasis is transmitted by the bites of the tsetse fly. It is uncommon among travellers but may occur in those who have been on game safaris. It occurs in scattered areas of Africa between the Sahara and the southern African countries. There may be a trypanosomal 'chancre' at the site of the bite and a febrile illness occurs. This may then be followed by a meningoencephalitis with central nervous or psychiatric symptoms and signs with the ultimate development of the classical picture of sleeping sickness.

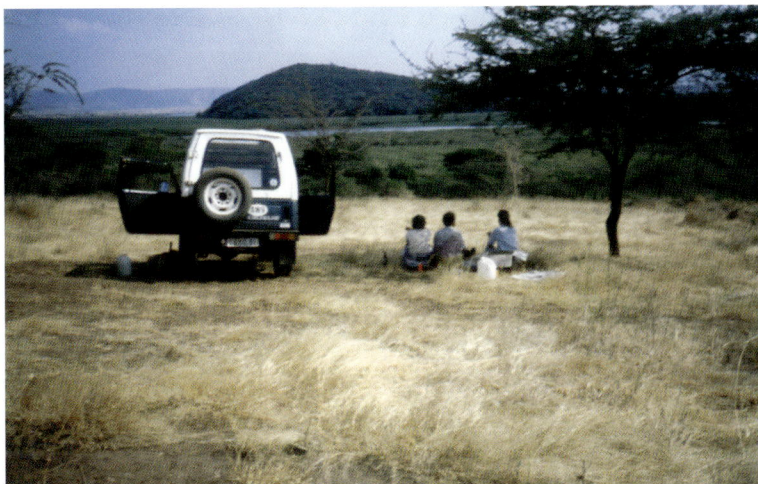

Dr Steve Mellor

Trypanosomiasis is a rare hazard for travellers on game safaris

■ *South American trypanosomiasis* is transmitted by the bites of bugs which inhabit cracks in the walls of adobe houses and emerge at night. It is very uncommon among travellers. The initial febrile illness may be followed after a long interval by paralytic lesions of smooth muscle leading to dilatation of hollow organs such as the oesophagus, large intestine or heart.

Tick-borne diseases

■ *Tick typhus* is caused by infection with Rickettsia organisms transmitted by tick bites. It occurs in African countries. A necrotic eschar forms at the site of the bite and a febrile illness with lymphadenopathy and possibly a rash and splenomegaly occurs. There is no reliable early diagnostic test but at a later stage serological tests may be carried out.

■ *Lyme disease* is caused by Borrelia burgdorferi transmitted by the bites of deer or sheep ticks. It has a widespread distribution which includes the UK, continental Europe and the USA. The tick bite may go unnoticed although there may be a rash (erythema chronicum migrans) which spreads out from the site of the bite. A flu-like illness follows with muscle and/or joint pains which may be followed by a persistent or relapsing illness with fatigue and joint pains. There may also be central nervous or cardiac involvement.

■ *Tick-borne encephalitis* is found chiefly in forested areas of northern and eastern Europe and Scandinavia. It may be suspected in unvaccinated travellers who have been on walking holidays in such areas and who have had tick bites or, for example, who have been exposed to bites by wearing shorts.

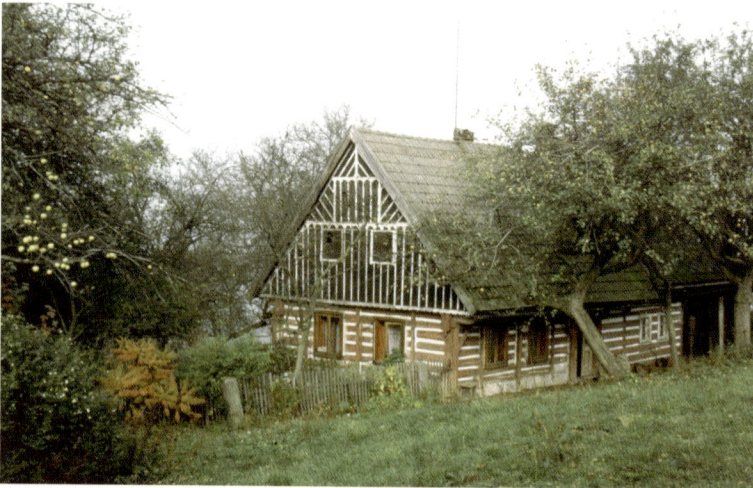

Dr M Townend

Tick-borne encephalitis is a possible hazard of walking in the forests of Eastern Europe

Hepatitis

- **Hepatitis A** is the most common 'immunisable' infectious disease likely to be acquired by travellers to countries which have relatively low standards of food, water or general hygiene. It is acquired by the faecal/oral route from contaminated food or water. Early symptoms are malaise, lethargy, anorexia and nausea, followed after a few days by jaundice. Often the patient feels better by the time jaundice develops. Fulminant hepatitis may occur but is not common. In confirming the diagnosis, the white cell count may be normal or reduced, liver function tests will show marked elevation of transaminase levels and serological tests will be positive.

- **Hepatitis B** presents in a similar way but usually after a longer incubation period and with a greater tendency to rashes and joint pains. There may be a history of exposure to risk by means of medical or surgical treatment involving invasive techniques including injections, blood transfusion, body piercing, tattooing or sexual contact. The likelihood of hepatitis B is greater in long-term travellers and expatriates who have been exposed to risk for longer periods. Diagnosis is made in a similar manner to that of hepatitis A, great care being necessary when taking and handling blood specimens from these and all patients suspected of having any form of hepatitis. Fulminant hepatitis may occasionally follow and hepatoma is a possible long-term consequence.

- **Other forms of hepatitis.** Hepatitis C is the most common cause of non-A, non-B hepatitis and, like hepatitis B, it is a blood-borne infection. It may lead to fulminant hepatitis and carries a higher risk of chronic liver disease and hepatoma. Hepatitis E is a faecal/oral infection which is found in the Indian subcontinent and also in parts of Africa and the Far East.

Viral haemorrhagic fevers

Dengue is the most widespread cause of haemorrhagic fever but other viral infections such as Lassa, Marburg and Ebola viruses have gained much greater notoriety. They appear to have originated as infecting agents in non-human mammals in some African countries but can be transmitted from human to human, especially by contact with body fluids. They are usually characterised by fever, headache and sore throat and the patient rapidly becomes prostrated by an obviously severe illness. There may then be abdominal symptoms, musculoskeletal pains, rash and evidence of bleeding in the skin and elsewhere. Admission to a specialised unit is required for patients who have visited an African country and are suspected of this type of illness.

Diseases caused by flukes

■ **Schistosomiasis** is acquired by penetration of intact human skin by cercarial larvae of Schistosoma shed by freshwater snails. Eggs are deposited in or near water in human faeces and hatch into miracidia which infect the snails. Larvae mature in the human liver

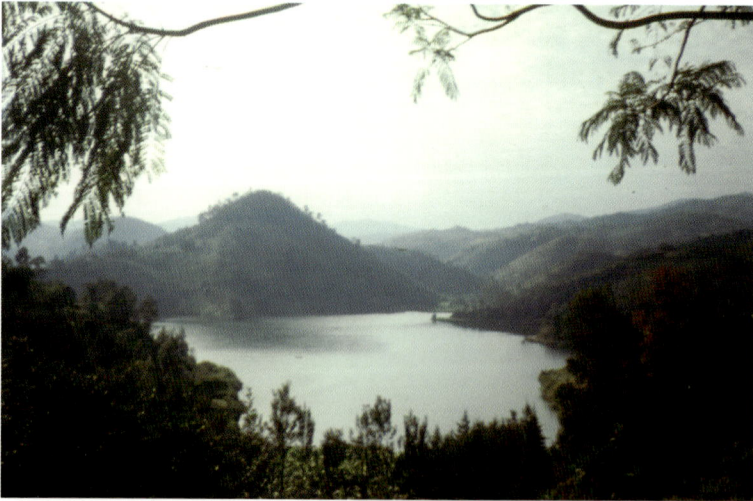

Lake Kivu, Rwanda – swimming in African lakes is likely to lead to infection with schistosomiasis

and migrate to mesenteric veins in the case of S. mansoni and S. japonicum and vesical veins in the case of S. haematobium where they may exist as a male/female pair for several years. During this time they produce ova which may cause intense granulomatous reaction in the bowel or bladder.

An itchy papular rash known as swimmer's itch may occur following skin penetration. Subsequently there may be a febrile reaction known as Katayama fever, with eosinophilia and possibly gastrointestinal symptoms, cough and wheezing or splenomegaly. Granuloma formation in the bowel leads to a dysenteric illness with diarrhoea and the passage of blood, intestinal ulceration and pseudopolyposis. In the bladder there is pseudopapilloma formation and haematuria and in the long-term obstructive uropathy and carcinoma of the bladder may occur.

The disease may be suspected in a traveller who has visited Africa or the Far East or possibly South America and who has swum, bathed or waded in fresh (ie non-salt) water. Diagnosis may be suspected by finding eosinophilia and confirmed by finding eggs in the urine or stools, by rectal biopsy or by serological tests. Treatment is usually by praziquantel.

Diseases of close personal contact

▪ **Tuberculosis** is unlikely to be acquired by travellers unless they are exposed to increased risk by virtue of having spent prolonged periods in close physical contact with local residents in countries with a high level of endemicity. Health-care workers, teachers, other aid workers and long-term expatriates are most at risk. Symptoms in the traveller will be similar to those seen in other tuberculous presentations and may include fever, weight-loss, sweating, malaise and cough. The polymorphonuclear leucocyte count is usually normal but may be reduced in the case of miliary or widely disseminated disease.

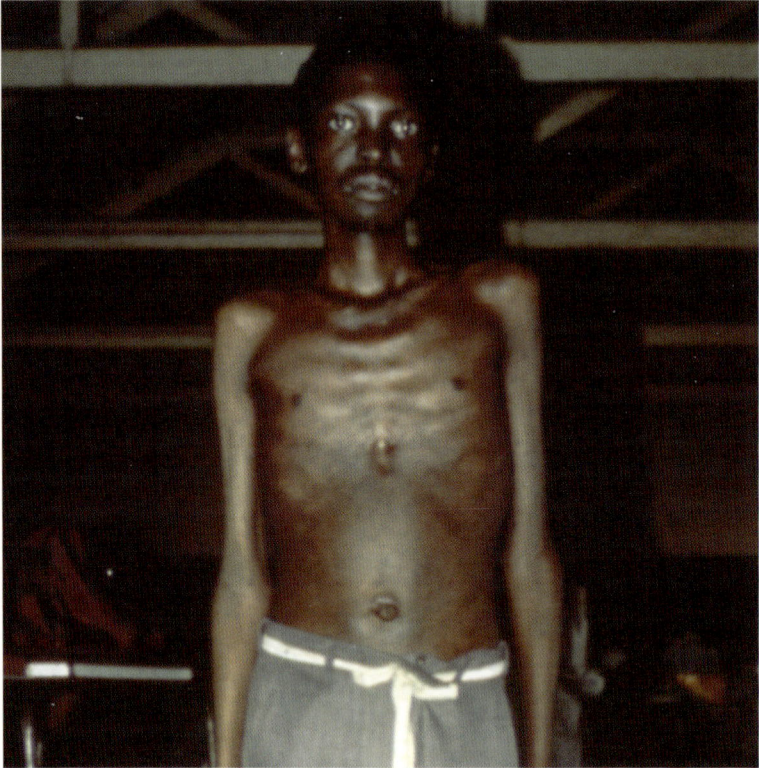

Wellcome Tropical Medicine Resource and SB Lucas

Tuberculosis is a hazard of close personal contact in many countries

■ *Meningococcal* infection is usually a rapidly developing illness with septicaemia and meningitis but it could possibly be seen early in its course in a returning traveller. The travellers most at risk are the same as the at-risk groups for tuberculosis but a majority of those who develop meningococcal infection are under the age of 25.

■ *Diphtheria* is also relatively unlikely to occur in travellers and is most likely to occur in the same high risk categories as tuberculosis and meningococcal infection. In addition, it may be suspected in travellers who have visited countries previously forming part of the Soviet Union. The typical illness with fever and sore throat with membrane formation may be seen but diphtheria may also present as a skin ulcer with a sloughing base. Diphtheria responds well to penicillin but admission to a specialist unit will be required as diphtheria toxin may have serious neurological or cardiological consequences.

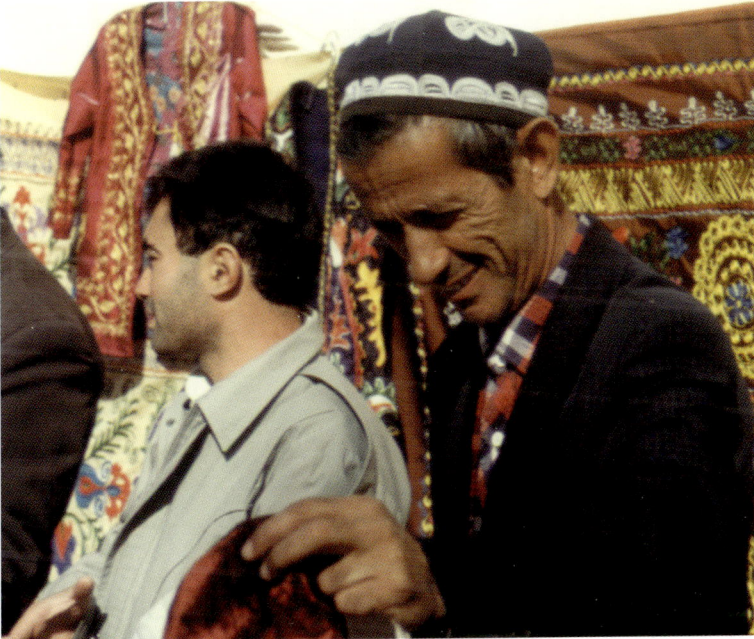

Dr M Townend

In an Uzbek market – diptheria is now a hazard of close personal contact in many former Soviet countries

Rabies

Symptomatic rabies is fortunately rare among returning travellers and is invariably fatal. More commonly a traveller may present on returning home with a history of a bite, scratch or lick from a dog or other mammal such as a monkey. Rabies is present in all countries outside the UK, Ireland, Norway, Sweden, Japan, Australia, New Zealand and parts of Malaysia and other Far East countries. The highest risk is present in the Indian subcontinent, Thailand and South America. Post-exposure vaccination is needed in all travellers who have been bitten, scratched or licked in a country where there is a risk of rabies. Pre-exposure vaccination reduces the number of doses of post-exposure vaccination needed.

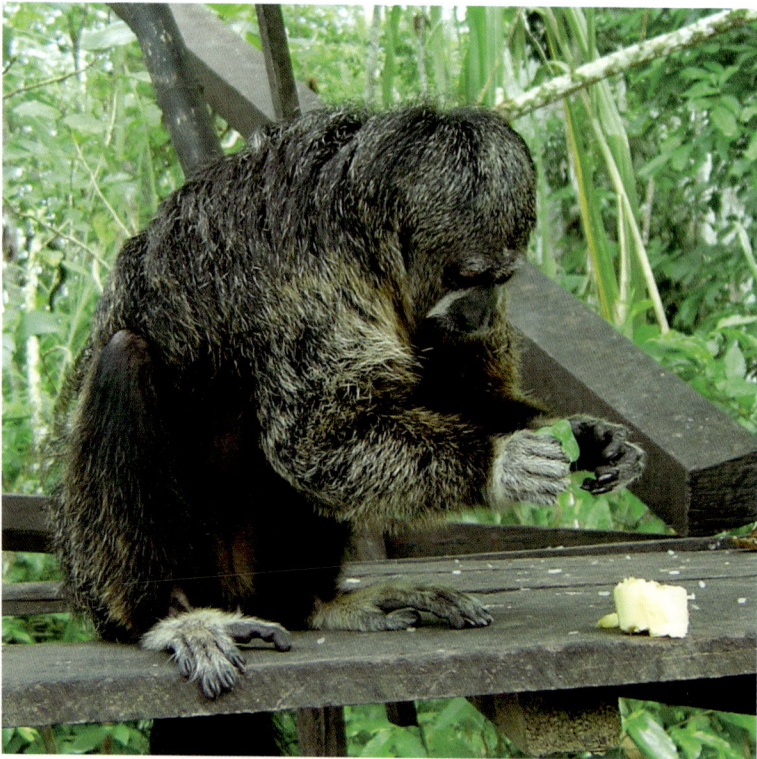

Dr M Townend

While dogs are common vectors for rabies, other small mammals such as monkeys can be implicated

Legionella

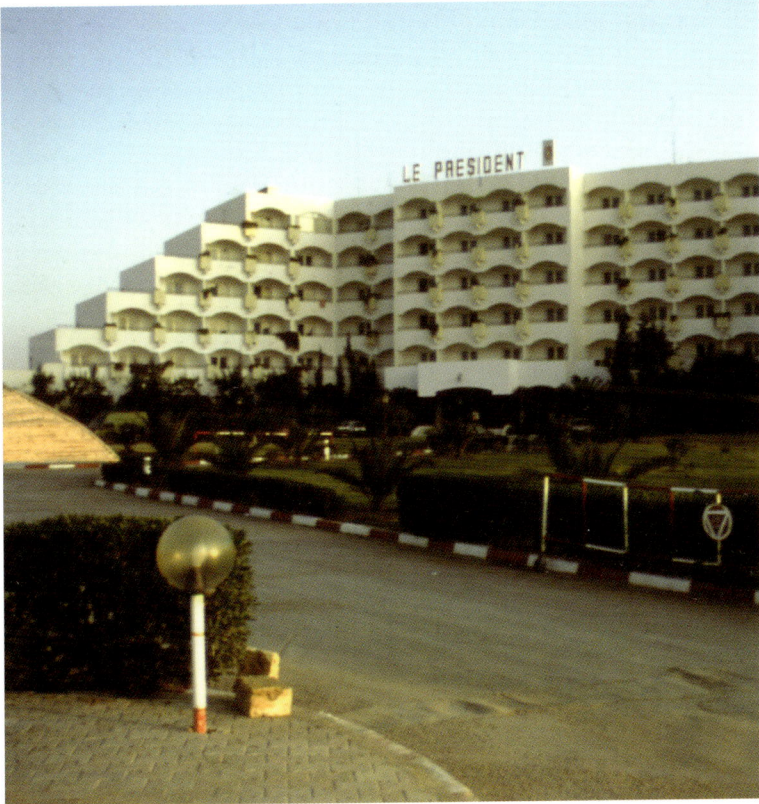

Air-conditioning and showers in hotels may be responsible for infection with Legionella

Legionella infection is acquired by inhalation of water droplets containing L. pneumophila. The bacteria have a preference for warm water and tend to multiply in water tanks on hotel roofs, from which they may contaminate the air-conditioning system, and in shower heads and spa pools. Illness is more likely to occur in the elderly or in travellers who are immunocompromised by drugs or disease. It should therefore be suspected as a cause of pneumonia in such travellers but as the infection causes multi-organ disease it should also be considered in the differential diagnosis of other conditions such as diarrhoea. It is usually treated with erythromycin.

Sexually transmitted diseases

▓ HIV/AIDS

Many travellers have sexual encounters while abroad. They may be planned, as in the case of so-called 'sex tourists' who travel with sexual adventure as a prime objective, or casual or opportunistic in the case of many other travellers. In Africa and, to a lesser extent, South America and the Caribbean, HIV infection has become very widespread through heterosexual contact, perinatal transmission and infected blood transfusions. In Asia it is spreading ever more rapidly by transmission from infected travellers, imported blood products and, increasingly, from 'core groups' of prostitutes and injecting drug users and their sexual partners. In Western Europe, North America and Australasia the chief routes of transmission are by homosexual and bisexual men, injecting drug users and, increasingly, heterosexual contact. Casual or planned sexual encounters, whether homosexual or heterosexual, with previously unknown partners carry a great risk, especially if safe sex, ie non-penetrative or with the use of condoms, has not been practiced. In particular, there is a high rate of HIV infection among workers in the 'sex industry' in tourist areas, eg in Thailand and other Southeast Asian countries where sex tourism is common.

Travellers may return home worried about the risk of infection with HIV from sexual contact or from invasive medical treatment, procedures such as body piercing or tattooing or sharing needles when taking injected drugs. Blood should be taken for serological investigation after counselling, bearing in mind that seroconversion may not occur for up to three months after exposure to infection, and re-testing may be necessary after three months. Testing for hepatitis B should also be considered. Sexual behaviour and exposure to the other modes of transmission should be included in the history taken from returning travellers and, if a traveller who has been at risk from HIV infection presents with a fever, the possibility of a seroconversion reaction should be considered and testing done. Specialist referral will be needed if a positive test is found.

■ *Other STDs*

It is beyond the scope of this brief guide to give a detailed account of the many other sexually transmitted diseases which are still widespread and tend to be forgotten in the anxiety about HIV. Syphilis and gonorrhoea are relatively common in developing countries and may still be encountered in some other areas, especially among prostitutes. Chlamydia infection is also widespread, as is genital herpes. Chancroid, lymphogranuloma venereum and granuloma inguinale are frequently found in developing countries.

Symptoms which should arouse suspicion and trigger referral to a department of Genitourinary Medicine include:
- ■ Penile or vaginal discharge
- ■ Herpetic genital lesions or warts
- ■ Penile or vulval sores or ulcers
- ■ Swellings with or without ulceration in the groin or genital areas
- ■ Rashes

BIBLIOGRAPHY

The following books provide useful reference material on the diseases referred to in this chapter:
1. Bell DR (ed). Lecture Notes on Tropical Medicine (4th ed).
    Oxford: Blackwell Science, 1995
2. Cook GC, Zumla AI (eds). Manson's Tropical Diseases (21st ed). Edinburgh:
    Elsevier Science, 2003
3. Travel Medicine and Migrant Health. Lockie C, Walker E, Calvert L, Cossar J, Knill-Jones R,
    Raeside F (eds). London: Churchill Livingstone, 2000 (2nd ed in preparation)
4. DuPont HL, Steffen R. Textbook of Travel Medicine and Health.
    Hamilton: BC Decker Inc., 2001
5. Dawood R (ed). Travellers' Health: How to Stay Healthy Abroad (4th ed).
    Oxford: Oxford University Press, 2002
6. Townend M, Howell K. Travel Health for the Primary Care Team.
    Dinton: Quay Books, 1999
7. Arya OP, Hart CA (eds). Sexually Transmitted Infections and AIDS in the Tropics.
    Wallingford: CAB International, 1998
8. Harries AD, Maher D, Raviglione MC, Chaulet P, Nunn PP, van Praag E. TB/HIV:
    A Clinical Manual. Geneva: World Health Organisation, 1996
9. Ericsson CD, DuPont HL, Steffen R. Travelers; Diarrhea. Hamilton: BC Decker Inc., 2003
10. Schalgenhauf P. Travelers' Malaria. Hamilton: BC Decker Inc., 2001

CHAPTER FOUR

Practical points in management

Useful drugs and doses

It is not intended to provide a complete travel medicine formulary here but to list some of the more common medications which may be of use in managing returned travellers.

Antibacterial drugs

- **Ciprofloxacin** is a broad spectrum quinolone which is active against most of the intestinal bacterial pathogens in an oral dose of 500mg twice a day. It is usually given for 5 to 7 days but there is evidence that a single dose of 500mg may be effective against travellers' diarrhoea. It is not recommended for children but may be given if necessary in a daily dose of 7.5-15mg/kg in two divided doses. In adult travellers with acute and frequent diarrhoea of more than 24-48 hours duration with fever it is reasonable to give ciprofloxacin empirically while awaiting the result of a stool culture. Resistance of enteric organisms to ciprofloxacin is beginning to be seen in some areas.

- **Azithromycin** is a macrolide which may be used in a dose of 500mg daily for 3 days to treat infections with ciprofloxacin-resistant enteric organisms.

- **Tetracyclines** are effective against Borrelia burgdorferi, the causative organism in Lyme disease. They are all more or less equivalent in action and are given orally. Oxytetracycline 250-500mg 6-hourly has the virtue of cheapness while doxycycline is taken only once a day in a dose of 100-200mg but is more expensive. If the characteristic erythema chronicum migrans is seen around a tick bite it is reasonable to start treatment with a tetracycline. Tetracyclines are not recommended for children and pregnant women as they are deposited in growing teeth and bones.

■ **Erythromycin** is a macrolide antibiotic which is effective against Legionella pneumophila, the causative organism in Legionnaire's disease. It is usually given in an oral dose of 500mg 6-hourly and should be considered for any traveller with an atypical lower respiratory tract infection, especially the elderly or immunocompromised.

■ **Flucloxacillin** is a penicillin which is effective against penicillinase producing staphylococci. It is useful for a variety of infected skin lesions including secondarily infected insect bites in an oral dose of 250-500mg 6-hourly in adults. In children under the age of 2 years the dose is one quarter of the adult dose and in children between 2 and 10 years it is half the adult dose.

Malaria treatment regimens

It is not the intention here to describe drug regimens for prophylaxis of malaria but for treatment only. The primary care team will not usually be involved in treating malaria but may encounter a traveller who has started of his own accord or on medical advice on a treatment course of antimalarial drugs prior to returning home. In areas where drug prophylaxis is a problem it is not unusual for a long-term or remote traveller to carry a treatment course rather than taking prophylaxis.

The following regimens are recommended for malaria treatment in the UK:

1. **Quinine:** 600mg 8-hourly orally for 7 days
   followed by
   Fansidar: 3 tablets as a single dose
   OR
   Tetracycline: 250mg 6-hourly for 7 days

   This is a suitable regimen for falciparum malaria in adults. Severely ill adults need to be admitted to hospital for intravenous quinine therapy. *Mefloquine* (20-25mg/kg, maximum dose 1.5Gm, either as a single dose or preferably in 2-3 divided doses 6 to 8-hourly) or *halofantrine* (rarely used because of potential cardiac effects) may be used instead of quinine.

2. *Malarone (atovaquone + proguanil):* 4 tablets once daily for 3 days

This is also a suitable regimen for falciparum malaria in adults.

3. *Chloroquine:* an initial oral dose of 600mg for adults followed by a further dose of 300mg after 6-8 hours and 300mg daily for 2 days

This regimen is used for the more benign forms of malaria but in the case of P. vivax and P. ovale it should be followed by:

Primaquine: 15mg daily for adults for 14-21 days to eliminate the dormant liver stage in vivax or ovale malaria

This should not be used during pregnancy although initial treatment with chloroquine is permissible.

Other antiprotozoal drugs

■ *Metronidazole* in an adult oral dose of 800mg 8-hourly for 5 days is effective against amoebiasis in its invasive dysenteric phase. The same dosage should be continued for up to 10 days in the case of amoebic liver abscess. For giardiasis a dose of 2g per day for 3 days is needed.

■ *Diloxanide* in an adult oral dose of 500mg 8-hourly for 10 days is used in the elimination of amoebic cysts in chronic amoebiasis or following treatment with metronidazole.

It is unlikely that the primary care team will be much involved with children's doses of the above drugs but they may be found in the British National Formulary (BNF).

Anthelmintic drugs

▪ **Mebendazole** is widely used in the UK for adults and children over the age of 2 years in a single dose of 100mg for threadworms. But it is also effective against whipworms and hookworms in a dose of 100mg twice a day for 3 days.

▪ **Piperazine** may be given as an elixir (adult dose 15ml daily for 7 days) or a powder with added senna (adult dose 1 sachet, repeated after 14 days) for threadworms. For roundworms the doses respectively are 30ml repeated after 14 days or 1 sachet repeated after a month. It has potentially more side effects than mebendazole.

▪ **Albendazole** is used for the treatment of hydatid disease in an adult oral dose of 800mg daily (divided) in cycles of 28 days of treatment with 14-day gaps, sometimes for prolonged periods. It is also used in the treatment of whipworms and strongyloidiasis in a dose of 400mg twice a day for 3 days.

▪ **Niclosamide** in an adult oral dose of 2g followed after 2 hours by a purgative such as senna is used to treat both beef and pork tapeworms and also the fish tapeworm Diphyllobothrium latum.

▪ **Thiabendazole** is given in an adult oral dose of 25mg/kg (max 1.5g) 12-hourly for 3 days in the treatment of strongyloidiasis. It may also be used to treat cutaneous larva migrans.

▪ **Praziquantel** is given in an adult oral dose of 40mg/kg in 2 divided doses 12 hours apart for the treatment of schistosomiasis. If a traveller returning from Africa has swum or waded in water and develops an itchy papular rash the drug may be given in anticipation of the diagnosis.

For children's doses of anthelmintics the British National Formulary (BNF) should be consulted.

Antidiarrhoeal drugs

■ **Loperamide** is a popular and relatively safe drug used by travellers to reduce stool frequency. The adult oral dose is 4mg initially followed by 2mg after each loose stool up to a maximum of 8mg daily. It may be continued for several days but it is important to pay attention to oral rehydration and not to rely on loperamide alone. The dose for children from 4-8 years is 1mg 3-4 times a day for no more than 3 days and from 9-12 years 2mg 3-4 times a day for up to 5 days. It is not recommended in children under 4 years.

■ **Codeine phosphate** and **co-phenotrope ('Lomotil')** are possible alternatives but they are not recommended for children and carry an increased risk of dependence or side-effects.

■ **Oral rehydration** may be achieved by the use of ready prepared sachets such as 'Dioralyte' or 'Rehidrat' or by using a solution of 5 teaspoons of sugar or glucose plus half a teaspoon of salt in one pint of water. It is the treatment of choice for acute diarrhoea.

Antihistamines

Antihistamine drugs are useful in the treatment of itchy, allergic skin rashes such as those seen in response to insect bites.

■ **Chlorpheniramine** is a cheap and long established antihistamine which may cause drowsiness. Its adult dose is 4mg 4 to 6-hourly. Children's doses are 1mg twice a day from 1-2 years, 1mg 4 to 6-hourly from 2-5 years, 2mg 4 to 6-hourly from 6-12 years.

■ **Loratadine** is a less sedative but more expensive alternative with the advantage of a once-a-day dosage, 10mg for adults and children over the age of 12 years or over 30kg weight and 5mg for children under 30kg.

Useful investigations

Haematology

■ *Polymorphonuclear leucocyte count:*
Normal range 2.0-7.5 x 109/L (40-60%).
Raised in most bacterial infections, septicaemia, borreliosis, amoebic liver abscess.
Low in malaria, miliary TB, brucellosis (some cases), visceral leishmaniasis.
Normal in viral infections, typhoid, Rickettsia infections, localised TB, toxoplasmosis, brucellosis (some cases), trypanosomiasis

■ *Lymphocyte count:*
Normal range 1.5-4.0 x 109/L (20-40%).
Raised in viral infections.

■ *Eosinophil count:*
Normal range 0.04-0.4 x 109/L (1.6%).
Raised in schistosomiasis, filariasis, larva migrans and worm infestations in general.

■ *Blood film*
Stained film for malaria (thick and thin), filariasis (timing of specimen according to type of Filaria), trypanosomiasis and borreliosis.
Dark ground for borreliosis.

Biochemistry

Liver function tests

- **Serum transaminases** are raised in any disease which causes hepatocellular jaundice such as hepatitis A or B, yellow fever or leptospirosis, often to extremely high levels. Normal levels are:
  - AST < 42IU/L
  - ALT < 47IU/L
  - GGT < 30IU/L

- **Serum alkaline phosphatase** is raised in any condition associated with obstructive (cholestatic) jaundice but may rise to some extent if a cholestatic element develops in any of the above conditions. Normal value:
  - ALP < 275IU/L

Urine tests

- **Urine culture** is needed if a urinary tract infection is suspected as a cause of pyrexia.

- **Urine microscopy** (centrifuged specimen) is needed if urinary schistosomiasis is suspected.

Stool tests

- **Stool culture** is indicated for any traveller with diarrhoea which does not begin to resolve within 24-48 hours of returning home, is associated with pyrexia or the passage of blood or is becoming worse rather than better.

- **Stool microscopy** is needed for diagnosis of amoebiasis (freshly passed stool), giardiasis (cysts usually present, may need more than one specimen) and schistosomiasis (centrifuged).

Serology

There is a bewildering variety of serological tests for infectious and tropical diseases, some of which are more helpful than others. It is wise to consult the laboratory and/or a specialist in infectious or tropical diseases about which tests are most likely to be helpful. Some of the diseases for which serological tests are available are:

- Hepatitis A
- Hepatitis B
- Leptospirosis
- Salmonella spp.
- Amoebiasis
- Schistosomiasis
- Yellow fever
- Dengue
- Filariais
- Typhus

BIBLIOGRAPHY

Useful information on drugs and investigations can be found in the following books:
1. British National Formulary. London: British Medical Association and Royal Pharmaceutical Society of Great Britain
2. Bell DR (ed). Lecture Notes on Tropical Medicine (4th ed). Oxford: Blackwell Science, 1995
3. Cook GC, Zumla AI (eds). Manson's Tropical Diseases (21st ed). Edinburgh: Elsevier Science, 2003
4. DuPont HL, Steffen R. Textbook of Travel Medicine and Health. Hamilton: BC Decker Inc., 2001
5. Arya OP, Hart CA (eds). Sexually Transmitted Infections and AIDS in the Tropics. Wallingford: CAB International, 1998
6. Ericsson CD, DuPont HL, Steffen R. Travelers; Diarrhea. Hamilton: BC Decker Inc., 2003
7. Schalgenhauf P. Travelers' Malaria. Hamilton: BC Decker Inc., 2001

CHAPTER FIVE

Emerging and re-emerging infections

'New' diseases gain a great deal of publicity in the news media and it is important for those advising travellers to know of their existence and to be able to suspect their presence in returned travellers.

Emerging infections are defined as those which have begun to exist, have been newly recognised or have appeared to become more significant within the last 20 years. Re-emerging infections are defined as those which have appeared to become more significant within the last 20 years after a period of relative quiescence.

Examples of emerging and re-emerging infection are given overleaf in Table 1.

It is not within the scope of this book to examine in detail all the emerging and re-emerging infections referred to in Table 1, but examples will be given with reference to some of the more recently emerging or re-emerging infections.

It will be obvious that in some of the examples used more than one mechanism may have played a part in the emergence of a disease.

How do infections emerge or re-emerge?

Novel infective agents

From time to time, an infection emerges which can be traced to an infective agent not previously recognised. A recent example of this is variant CJD (Creuzfeld-Jacob Disease).

Variant CJD (vCJD)

Although CJD had been known to exist for much longer it was only in 1996[1] that the new variant of the disease was recognised, occurring in much younger

Table 1

Emerging infections that do not appear to have existed previously:

- E. coli 0157
- HIV
- Human avian influenza.
- SARS
- Strains of staphylococci causing toxic shock syndrome
- Variant CJD

Newly identified emerging infections, with patterns of symptoms suggesting that they may have existed previously but have not been previously recognised:

- Campylobacter
- Cryptosporidium
- Hantavirus
- Hepatitis C
- Legionella
- Lyme disease
- Viral haemorrhagic fevers

Re-emerging infections:

- Cholera
- Dengue fever
- Diphtheria
- Malaria
- Tuberculosis

patients than the previously existing form of the disease and showing a slower rate of progression. Most of the cases reported to date have occurred in the United Kingdom where, in the late Eighties and early Nineties, bovine spongiform encephalopathy (BSE) had emerged with a rapid increase in incidence, peaking around 1992.

The clustering in place and time between these two diseases and their nature as progressive neurological conditions suggested an association and, in 1997, evidence emerged which suggested that they had a common causative agent[2]. BSE is one of the so-called transmissible spongiform encephalopathies – fatal diseases in animals characterised by the development of multiple cavities within the brain, and caused by the presence of a prion[3].

Prions are proteins which, unlike micro-organisms such as bacteria and viruses, do not contain any genetic material but are capable of bringing about damaging changes in other proteins. Probably the only previously recognised example of a human prion disease was kuru, whose effects included ataxia and dementia, seen only among highland dwellers in Papua New Guinea who honoured their dead by eating their brains. The disease ceased to exist following the ending of this practice.

The occurrence of vCJD thus represented the emergence of a novel infective agent for humans, with inter-species transmission (discussed later in this chapter) providing the vehicle for its entry into humans by the consumption of infected beef.

Bacterial or viral mutation

Micro-organisms which have previously existed and have not been pathogenic to humans may undergo changes which render them pathogenic, and organisms which have been pathogenic may undergo changes which make them more virulent. Escherchia coli has long had both commensal and pathogenic strains, but the emerging 0157 strain became more virulent by the acquisition of the ability to produce Shiga-like toxins[4].

Infection with this strain may lead to the development of bloody diarrhoea, thrombocytopaenia and haemolytic-uraemic syndrome. Staphylococci, while they are often present in symptomless carriers, are human pathogens. Some strains have acquired the ability to produce exotoxins responsible for the toxic shock syndrome[5], though the emergence of this syndrome has also been contributed to by host factors and human behaviour, ie the use of tampons for menstrual protection.

Since the advent of penicillin, staphylococci have also shown a remarkable ability to become resistant to antibiotics, culminating in the emergence of methicillin resistant staphylococcus aureus (MRSA)[6].

Inter-species transmission

One of the longest recognised examples of inter-species transmission is yellow fever, which was originally an infection of primates which has since become transmissible to humans via mosquito vectors. It has been postulated that HIV infection may also have originated in primates. Hantavirus[7] in rodents has become transmissible to humans, resulting in the hantavirus pulmonary syndrome, and variant CJD has also succeeded in crossing the species barrier from cattle infected with BSE.

Avian influenza[8]

The most recent example of inter-species transmission which has achieved worldwide publicity is avian influenza. At the time of writing, outbreaks of avian influenza caused by the H5N1 viral strain in chickens had been reported in Vietnam and Thailand, with cases also reported in Japan, Taiwan, China and South Korea. A total of 14 cases of human infection had been reported in Thailand and Vietnam at the time of writing, with 11 deaths.

The infection is not directly transmissible between humans, and is only infrequently transmitted to humans from chickens. The human cases reported in the current outbreaks had all had close contact with chickens, probably acquiring infection via inhalation of particles of chicken faecal material. Rapid culling of poultry appears to be the most effective means of controlling the spread of infection and, while there is no evidence that infection can be acquired, the European Union acted quickly to ban the import of chicken products from Thailand.

Although avian influenza is not currently transmissible between humans it could become a major threat to human health in the future by virtue of two well-established properties of influenza viruses.

The first is their ability to mutate. The so-called antigenic shift – mutations in surface antigens in influenza viruses – is responsible for the changes that occur from year to year in influenza viruses necessitating the incorporation of new strains into each year's current influenza vaccine.

The second important property is the ability of viruses to exchange genetic material between different strains. It is possible that if avian influenza infection were acquired by an individual already infected with a human influenza virus, the avian virus could acquire genetic material from the human virus enabling it to become transmissible between humans.

As avian influenza appears to be particularly virulent in humans this could represent a significant threat to human health comparable to the 'Spanish flu' pandemic in 1918 which was responsible for more deaths than The Great War of 1914 to 1918.

Inter-species transmission of a different kind may also increase the likelihood of human transmission of avian influenza if passage through pigs takes place, rendering the virus more easily transmissible to humans.

Environmental factors

Climate changes, whether long-term as a result of global warming due to human activity, or shorter term as a result of natural phenomena such as El Niño, may be favourable to the growth of micro-organisms or the presence of vectors. For example, an increase in ambient temperature and/or an increase in rainfall may increase the likelihood of favourable breeding conditions for mosquitoes, leading to the emergence or re-emergence of infections such as malaria and dengue in regions where they have not previously occurred or from which they had previously been eradicated.

Host factors

In addition to changes in the pathogenicity of staphylococci the preference of many women for using tampons rather than any other type of menstrual protection is an example of a host factor which has created an environment favourable to the growth of these newly-emerged strains.

Human behaviour

The earliest conditions favouring transmission of disease as a result of human behaviour probably arose in the change from the nomadic hunter-gatherer lifestyle to settled agriculture and ultimately to urbanisation. Irrigation and the damming of watercourses for drinking water provided breeding grounds for mosquitoes, and urbanisation resulted in favourable conditions for person-to-person transmission of infection. Trade and imperial conquests created routes for the spread of infections from one part of the world to another.

HIV/AIDS

In more recent times, a combination of the above factors, together with easier and more rapid travel and sexual and drug-taking behaviour, resulted in a rapid spread of HIV infection throughout the world following its emergence[9]. At the time of writing, the UNAIDS database[10] estimated that as many as 60 million people worldwide could be infected with the HIV virus.

Although the syndrome of AIDS was first recognised in the western world in young homosexual men in the early Eighties, it rapidly became apparent that heterosexual contact was a major means of transmission, particularly in African countries[11] where it frequently appeared to be transmitted along major routes of travel. A high incidence of infection has also been found among commercial sex workers, their families and clients and among intravenous drug users. Vertical transmission from mother to child[12] is also a major means of transmission in many countries.

Human behaviour has thus been a major factor in the emergence and spread of HIV infection, and travel health advisers have a responsibility to warn all travellers of the possible consequences of sexual and drug-taking behaviour and invasive medical procedures.

The advent of HIV infection has also played a major role in the re-emergence of tuberculosis[13] as a global health problem. In addition, difficulty of ensuring adherence to treatment regimes has led to the emergence of multi-drug resistant tuberculosis.

Travel

The importance of travel in the spread of infection has been recognised throughout history, with trade and mass population movements in times of war and famine playing a major part. More recently, the ease and rapidity of modern transport has greatly facilitated the movement of immigrants, refugees and economic migrants as well as tourists and business travellers. In turn, this has facilitated the rapid spread of both existing and emerging and re-emerging infections.

In practices with large populations of immigrants or ethnic minority UK residents there is a likelihood that members of the immigrant community may have brought with them diseases such as tuberculosis. Ethnic minority UK residents visiting family or friends in their country of origin are also known to be at risk of returning with infections such as tuberculosis or malaria[14] and take fewer prophylactic measures than do other travellers to the same countries as they do not necessarily perceive that they are at risk.

Severe acute respiratory syndrome(SARS)

The emergence and spread of SARS demonstrates very well the role of modern travel in the emergence and spread of infection[15]. In February, 2003, a doctor from southern China arrived in Hong Kong. He had been unwell for a few days but rapidly deteriorated and was admitted to hospital in Hong Kong where he died. His brother-in-law, two nurses at the hospital and seven guests from the same floor of his hotel became ill. One hotel guest admitted to hospital transmitted the illness to 88 health care workers and 18 medical students and a patient discharged from hospital appears to have infected over 200 residents in a housing estate. All suffered a severe respiratory infection with atypical pneumonia.

By March, 2003, outbreaks of a similar illness were reported in Singapore, Vietnam and Toronto[16] which appeared to be connected with guests who had stayed at the hotel, and other clusters of cases were reported in connection with travellers who had recently visited southern China.

The origin of the infection appeared to have been the Guangdong province of China at the end of 2002, where over 300 cases and five deaths had occurred. Subsequently, cases were detected in other South East Asian countries, Japan and as far afield as Europe, the United States, South Africa and South America.

Eventually, the causative organism was identified as a type of coronavirus not previously identified[17]. Previously identified coronaviruses have been associated with less severe respiratory infections such as the common cold, and it seems likely that the new virus was a mutation. Although this was the primary reason for the emergence of SARS it is clear that travel was a major factor in its emergence and spread, and both national and international bodies issued guidelines for travellers to infected areas.

Political and economic factors

The influence of political and economic factors on public health measures can have an enormous impact on the re-emergence of previously controlled infections. There are two very good examples of this in recent history.

Malaria
In the early Sixties, malaria was almost eradicated from India. The eradication programme initially ran into difficulties because of shortages of DDT used to control mosquitoes. Later the programme experienced inadequate finance and both technical and administrative problems. The result was that malaria has since returned as a major public health problem[18]. Partial immunity develops by adulthood in those constantly exposed to infection but visitors to India continue to require malaria prophylaxis in all but the high altitude areas in the north of the country.

Diphtheria
Until the dissolution of the Soviet Union in the early Nineties, diphtheria was controlled by an immunisation programme. Following dissolution the Soviet Union was replaced by a large number of autonomous states without the financial, administrative and public health structures of the former superstate. As a result, immunisation programmes collapsed and diphtheria re-emerged as a threat to the health of the indigenous population[19].

Visitors from countries in which diphtheria is only a faint historical memory did not recognise it as a potential health threat and were also at risk if they were not adequately immunised.

Emerging infections of unknown origin

In 1991, cholera emerged in Peru[20] and, around the same time, cases were also reported in Ecuador and Chile. The outbreak began on the Pacific coast and although its origin is not entirely clear it is possible that it was the result of the discharge of sewage into the sea by a ship off the Pacific coast of Peru.

Whatever its original cause, infection spread rapidly to poor urban areas and the headwaters of the Amazon, resulting in widespread water-borne dissemination and the disease threatened to become endemic in Peru, with a consequent threat to the health of both indigenous people and travellers.

How do we recognise and track emerging and re-emerging diseases?

The first port of call for most patients in the UK is still the GP's practice. Individual clinicians need to be aware that previously unrecognised diseases may occur and that diseases thought to be under control in the UK may still be prevalent in other countries and may again become prevalent here. It is also important for them to be aware of the countries or regions where diseases are known to be emerging or re-emerging.

Recognition and reporting of symptoms which do not conform to recognised patterns or which suggest the re-emergence of a previously controlled disease are of the greatest importance in providing an early warning of an emerging or re-emerging disease. Medical journals play an important part by alerting readers to 'new' diseases or syndromes or to the resurgence of 'old' diseases. But electronic networks and databases may give a much more rapid early warning (see list of information sources on page 68).

National and international bodies such as the UK's Health Protection Agency, the American Centers for Disease Control and the World Health Organisation can greatly assist the dissemination of information by prompt recognition of occurrence and clustering of cases and investigation of suspected outbreaks. Surveillance of the progression of outbreaks and publication of data in forms readily accessible to all clinicians including the use of electronic networks are an important part of the work of such organisations.

The role of the GP and Practice Nurse in emerging and re-emerging infections

Awareness
GPs and practice nurses need to keep up-to-date with medical literature (and the national media!) and to consult appropriate websites frequently (see list of information sources on page 68).

Recognition
GPs and practice nurses need to be aware of the presenting symptoms of emerging or re-emerging infections and be prepared to suspect their presence. They should always enquire about recent travel as a routine part of history taking

Reporting
All patients with severe and/or unexplained symptoms should be referred or admitted to hospital for expert advice. Unexplained symptoms or suspected cases of emerging or re-emerging infections should be reported to the local Health Protection Agency, and reporting of notifiable diseases is a legal requirement for all clinicians.

Prevention
An individual risk assessment should be carried out for all travellers prior to travel and appropriate advice given. It is not adequate to give the same blanket pre-travel advice for all travellers to the same country, irrespective of the nature of their journey and activities, or to concentrate only on vaccinations as these can prevent only about 5% of all travel-related health risks. At least one member of any practice giving advice to travellers or seeing them on their return home should be trained in the medical problems of travel.

Useful information sources on emerging and re-emerging infections

(see also appendix II for an expanded list of information sources on travel-related health problems)

- **Health Protection Agency (England and Wales)**, www.hpa.org.uk

- **Scottish Centre for Infection and Environmental Health**, www.show.scot.nhs.uk/scieh

- **NaTHNaC** – The National Travel Health Network and Centre – based at the Hospital for Tropical Diseases. Advice line for healthcare professionals only: 020 7380 9234 (09.00-12.00 and 14.00-16.30, Monday to Friday)

- **World Health Organisation**, www.who.int/en

- **Centers for Disease Control (USA)**, www.cdc.gov

- **Travax Travel Health Database for Healthcare Professionals** (provides country-specific information and information and advice on a wide variety of travel-related health problems), www.travax.nhs.uk

- **Fit For Travel Database** (a public access website using information based on the Travax database), www.fitfortravel.scot.nhs.uk

- **Foreign and Commonwealth Office**, www.fco.gov.uk

- **OMNI** (provides links to sites giving information on disease outbreaks), www.omni.ac.uk/browse/mesh/detail/C0012652L0012652.html

- **TropNet Europ** (provides information on imported diseases in Europe), www.medwebplus.com/obj/3800

- **ProMED** (provides email information day by day to registered users on disease outbreaks worldwide), www.promedmail.org

- **VIS Online** (provides country specific information on outbreaks and an A-Z on each vaccine), www.apmsd.co.uk

REFERENCES

1. Will RG, Ironside JW, Zeidler M et al. A new variant of Creutzfeld-Jacob disease in the UK. Lancet, 1996. 347(9006): 921-5,

2. Bruce ME, Will RG, Ironside JW et al. Transmissions to mice indicate that "new variant" CJD is caused by the BSE agent. Nature, 1997. 389(6650): 498-501

3. Prusiner SB. The prion diseases. Scientific American website (accessed 31.01.04) http://www.sciam.com/article.cfm?articleID=0009FD80-C3C6-1C5A-B882809EC588ED9F

4. Feng P, Lampel KA, Karch H, Whittam TS. Genotypic and phenotypic changes in the emergence of Escherichia coli O157:H7. Journal of Infectious Diseases, 1998. 177(6): 1750-3

5. Wager GP. Toxic shock syndrome: a review. American Journal of Obstetrics and Gynecology. 1983. 146(1): 93-102

6. MRSA fact sheet. Centers for Disease Control and Prevention website (accessed 31.01.04) http://www.cdc.gov/ncidod/hip/Aresist/mrsafaq.htm

7. Doyle TJ, Bryan RT, Peters CJ. Viral hemorrhagic fevers and hantavirus infections in the Americas. Infectious Disease Clinics of North America, 1998. 12(1): 95-110

8. Avian influenza A(H5N1) - update 15, World Health Organisation website (accessed 02.02.04). http://www.who.int/csr/don/2004_02_02/en/

9. UNAIDS/World Health Organisation Global HIV/AIDS Global Database (accessed 02.02.04) http://www.who.int/GlobalAtlas/home.asp

10. Mansell PW. Acquired immune deficiency syndrome, leading to opportunistic infections, Kaposi's sarcoma, and other malignancies. Critical Reviews in Clinical Laboratory Sciences, 1984. 20(3): 191-204

11. Piot P, Quinn TC, Taelman H et al. Acquired immunodeficiency syndrome in a heterosexual population in Zaire. Lancet, 1984. 2(8394): 65-9

12. Fowler MG. Update: transmission of HIV-1 from mother to child. Current Opinion in Obstetrics and Gynecology, 1997. 9(6): 343-8

13. Drobniewski FA, Pozniak AL, Uttley AH. Tuberculosis and AIDS. Journal of Medical Microbiology, 1995. 43(2): 85-91

14. Behrens R. Travel morbidity on ethnic minority travellers. In Travel-Associated Disease. London: Royal College of Physicians, 1995

15. Chan-Yeung M, Yu WC. Outbreak of severe acute respiratory syndrome in Hong Kong Special Administrative Region: case report. BMJ 2003; 326: 850-52

16. Poutanen SM, Low DE, Henry B et al. Identification of severe acute respiratory syndrome in Canada. New England Journal of Medicine 2003 (accessed 02.02.04): http://content.nejm.org/cgi/content/abstract/NEJMoa030634v3

17. Ksiazek TG, Erdman D, Godsmith CS et al. A novel coronavirus associated with severe acute respiratory syndrome. New England Journal of Medicine 2003: http://content.nejm.org/cgi/content/abstract/NEJMoa030781v3

18. Sharma VP. Re-emergence of malaria in India. Indian Journal of Medical Research, 1996. 103: 26-45

19. Anon. Update: diphtheria epidemic – New Independent States of the Former Soviet Union. Morbidity & Mortality Weekly Report, 1996. 45(32): 693-7

20. Gotuzzo E, Cieza J, Estremadoyro L, Seas C. Cholera. Lessons from the epidemic in Peru. Infectious Disease Clinics of North America, 1994. 8(1): 183-205

APPENDIX I

A questionnaire for the returned traveller

This questionnaire may be completed by the traveller who consults a medical adviser or it may be used as the basis for taking a history.

1. **What countries did you visit on your most recent trip and how long did you stay in each?**

Country	Length of stay
1.	....
2.	....
3.	....
4.	....
5.	....
6.	....

2. **What other countries have you visited in the last 12 months and when were you there?**

   ....

3. **On what date did you leave home?**

   ....

4. **On what date did you return?**

   ....

5. **What kind of accommodation did you stay in?**

Western-style hotels.. ☐

Local-style hotels .... ☐

Lodges or other simple accommodation.............................. ☐

Staying with local people in their homes............................. ☐

Camping .... ☐

6. **What means of travel did you use during your journey?**

Air .... ☐

Sea .... ☐

River or lake boats... ☐

Rail (tourist or first class) .... ☐

Rail (basic).. ☐

Road (private or hired vehicles) .... ☐

Road (public transport) .... ☐

On foot .... ☐

7. **What was the purpose of your journey?**

Holiday.. ☐

Business .... ☐

Visiting relatives.. ☐

Working abroad.. ☐

Aid work with local people... ☐

Other (Please specify) ....

....

8. **Did you take antimalarial drugs?**

....

9. If so, did you take them for the full course as advised?

    ....

10. Did you take precautions against insect bites such as insect repellents, covering your skin or using a mosquito net?

    ....

11. Did you drink water (other than bottled water) which was not boiled, filtered or chemically purified?

    ....

12. Did you have ice in drinks?

    ....

13. Did you eat in cheap local restaurants or from street stalls?

    ....

14. Did you eat food which was not freshly cooked or from buffets?

    ....

15. Did you eat seafood?

    ....

16. Did you drink unboiled milk or eat dairy products (including butter, cheese or ice cream)?

    ....

17. Did you eat unpeeled fruit?

    ....

18. Did you swim anywhere other than in a purified swimming pool or wade through water or mud?

    ....

19. Did you ever go barefoot or wear flip-flops?

    ....

20. Were you bitten, scratched or licked by an animal?

    ....

21. **Did you walk through bush, grassland or forests wearing shorts?**

   ....

22. **Did you have sexual contact with local people or fellow travellers?**

   ....

23. **Did you have any medical treatment while abroad?**

   ....

24. **If so, did it involve injections, dressings, stitches, blood transfusions or operations?**

   ....

25. **Did you have any tattoos or body piercing done while abroad?**

   ....

26. **Did you have any of the following symptoms while abroad?**

   Diarrhoea.. ☐

   Vomiting... ☐

   Abdominal pain... ☐

   Raised temperature.. ☐

   Skin rash.. ☐

   Jaundice.. ☐

   Insect bites... ☐

   Tick bites.. ☐

27. **What vaccinations did you have before travelling?**

   1. ....   5. ....

   2. ....   6. ....

   3. ....   7. ....

   4. ....   8. ....

APPENDIX II

Useful information sources

Books

Dawood R. *Travellers' Health: How To Stay Healthy Abroad.*
Oxford: Oxford University Press 1992

Walker E, Williams G, Raeside F. *ABC Of Healthy Travel.*
London: BMJ Publishing Group 1993

Bell DR. *Lecture Notes On Tropical Medicine.*
Oxford: Blackwell Science Ltd 1995

British National Formulary, *Health Information For Overseas Travel (The Yellow Book).*
London: HMSO

Computer databases

Travax online database
Maintained by the Scottish Centre for Infection and Environmental Health
Tel: 0141 300 1100 or from www.travax.nhs.uk

Traveller database
Information from www.travellersoftware.co.uk or tel: 0114 279 7411

Exodus database
Information from www.exodus.ie

VIS Online
Information from www.apmsd.co.uk

Sources of information for health care professionals

Malaria Reference Laboratory
Public advice line: 09065 508908 (24-hour access, premium rate line)
Health care professionals: 020 7636 3924

Communicable Disease Surveillance Centre
61 Colindale Avenue, London NW9 5EQ
Health care professionals: 020 8200 6868

Hospital for Tropical Diseases Travel Clinic
Mortimer Market, Capper Street, Tottenham Court Road, London WC1E 6AU
Travellers' Healthline Advisory Service: 09061 337733 (premium rate line);
faxback service 09061 991992
Health care professionals: 020 7387 9300 or 4411
Website: www.thehtd.org

Liverpool School of Tropical Medicine
Public enquiry line: 0906 708 8807 (premium rate line)
Health care professionals: 0151 708 9393
Website: www.liv.ac.uk/lstm

Department of Infection & Tropical Medicine
Birmingham Heartlands Hospital
Health care professionals: 0121 766 6611

Department of Infectious Diseases & Tropical Medicine
North Manchester General Hospital
Health care professionals: 0161 720 2730

NaTHNaC – the National Travel Health Network and Centre
Based at the Hospital for Tropical Diseases, London, NaTHNaC has been set
up to develop and disseminate consistent national guidance on travel health, to
carry out surveillance of travel health hazards, to facilitate training in travel
health and to define research priorities. It will also take over the administration
of yellow fever vaccination centres. Advice line for health care professionals
only: 020 7380 9234 (09.00-12.00 and 14.00-16.30, Monday to Friday)

Health Protection Agency (England & Wales)
Website: www.hpa.org.uk

Scottish Centre for Infection and Environmental Health
Clifton House, Clifton Place, Glasgow G3 7LN
Tel: 0141 300 1100
Website: www.show.scot.nhs.uk/scieh

ProMED
Provides information by email about disease outbreaks
Website: www.promedmail.org

VIS Online
Provides reliable information on travel issues, country recommendations, malaria and outbreaks. It also gives comprehensive information on the full range of Aventis Pasteur MSD vaccines
Website: www.apmsd.co.uk

Other useful websites

World Health Organisation
www.who.int/en

OMNI
Provides links to sites giving information on disease outbreaks
www.omni.ac.uk/browse/mesh/detail/C0012652L0012652.html

TropNet Europ
Provides information on imported diseases in Europe
http://medwebplus.com/obj/3800

Fit for travel
Public access website with information from the Travax database in a form suitable for use by the general public
www.fitfortravel.scot.nhs.uk

Foreign & Commonweealth Office
www.fco.gov.uk

MASTA
The Medical Advice Service for Travellers Abroad
www.masta.org

US Centers for Disease Control
Standard US travel information and advice
www.cdc.gov/travel

Travel Health Online
US travel information and advice
www.tripprep.com

Post travel debriefing and counselling services

Interhealth
157 Waterloo Road, London SE1 8US
Tel: 020 7902 9000
Website: www.interhealth.org.uk

Dr Mike Jones
Edinburgh International Health Centre
Elphinstone Wing, Carberry, Musselburgh EH21 8PW
Tel: 0131 653 6767
Email: michaelejones@doctors.org.uk

Index